CANTATA
&
THE EXTINCTION THERAPIST

TWO PLAYS BY CLEM MARTINI

CANTATA FOREWORD BY NAHEED K. NENSHI
EXTINCTION THERAPIST FOREWORD BY CHRISTINE BRUBAKER

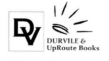

DURVILE &
UpRoute Books

Calgary, Alberta, Canada

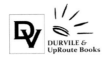

Durvile & UpRoute Books

UPROUTE IMPRINT OF DURVILE PUBLICATIONS LTD.

Calgary, Alberta, Canada
Durvile.com

Copyright © 2023 by Clem Martini

LIBRARY AND ARCHIVES CATALOGUING IN PUBLICATIONS DATA

Cantata & The Extinction Therapist: Two Plays by Clem Martini
Martini, Clem, author
Nenshi, Naheed K.; Cantata foreword
Brubaker, Christine; The Extinction Therapist foreword

1. Theatre | 2. Performing Arts | 3. Playwriting
4. Health Care Issues | 5 Mental Health Issues

978-1-990735-24-0 (pbk)
978-1-990735-38-7 (ebook)
978-1-990735-25-7 (audiobook)

Cover photograph, of Cantata: Cliff Kirschoff
Front cover photograph, Extinction Therapist: frame-work.ca
Photos of Cantata production: Cliff Kirschhoff
Book design: Lorene Shyba

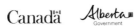

Durvile Publications would like to acknowledge the financial support of
The Government of Canada through the Canadian Heritage Canada Book Fund
and The Government of Alberta, Alberta Media Fund.
Printed in Canada. First edition, first printing. 2023.

Durvile Publications recognizes the traditional territories upon which our studios rest.
The Indigenous Peoples of Southern Alberta include the
Siksika, Piikani, and Kainai of the Blackfoot Confederacy; the Dene Tsuut'ina;
the Chiniki, Bearspaw, and Wesley Stoney Nakoda First Nations;
and the Region 3 Métis Nation of Alberta.

CANTATA

RUMOURS OF MY CRAZY, USELESS LIFE

FOREWORD BY NAHEED K. NENSHI

Dedicated to my family,
and to all the other
families struggling to
provide support
under difficult conditions.

ALSO BY CLEM MARTINI

The Comedian, 2019

The Untangling, with Olivier Martini, 2017

Upside Down:
A Family's Journey Through Mental Illness, 2015

The Ancient Comedians, 2014

Martini With A Twist:
An Anthology of Five Plays, 2012

Too Late, 2010

Bitter Medicine:
A Graphic Memoir of Mental Illness
with Olivier Martini, 2010

The Greek Playwright: What The Ancient Greeks
Have To Say To Contemporary Playwrights, 2009

The Blunt Playwright, 2006

The Judgment, 2006

The Plague, 2005

The Mob, 2004

Something Like A Drug:
An Oral History of Theatresports,
eds. Clem Martini, Kathleen Foreman, 1995

FOREWORD
NAHEED K. NENSHI

I SAW *Cantata: Rumours of My Crazy, Useless Life* in the most 2022 way possible. I had been so careful during the pandemic. I had to be a role model. Not only was I a public figure, I also lived with an 81-year-old roommate, my mother, and had to be responsible to her. I had worked so hard to not get Covid-19. But I was fully vaccinated, things were looking better, and I had the chance to travel for the first time in a couple of years for work. Of course, I ended up bringing the virus home.

My mother and I each spent a few days pretty sick with Covid. I was feeling much better, I was testing negative—past the infections phase—and it was closing night of the new Clem Martini play that I really wanted to see. So, I masked up, sat far away from everyone else, or as far away as I could in the sold-out crowd. There were a couple of seats set aside for people who wanted to isolate themselves from others, again, very 2022. And I sat down and watched the show.

I was surprised at my emotional reaction. It was clear from the first few minutes that this story was not going to have a happy ending. Or not a conventionally happy ending anyway. But more about that in a minute.

It put me in mind of Arthur Miller's *The Crucible:* the viewer can see what's going to happen and can feel the terrible momentum towards that end. But the viewer also knows there's nothing that can be done to stop it.

Nonetheless, there is beauty and intensity and humanity in hearing the story.

After the show, I wanted to leave quickly—with my mask on and all. But I also wanted to eavesdrop on the other audience members, to hear if they experienced what I did. Plus, my hands were shaking, and I wasn't sure I could drive quite yet. I ran into Brian Jensen, who played Dennis, outside on a lovely spring evening. I congratulated him on his performance, and he said that it was a great honour to be in the show, but he was glad the run was over. "It's just hard," he said. "I live in the character, but I also cry as someone hearing the story."

People often ask me why I love the theatre as much as I do. One of the answers I give is that it is always remarkable for me to experience art in the moment of its creation. Unlike, say, a painting that we can look at centuries after it was made, the play is made as we watch it. No two performances are the same. But a brilliantly written play, like this one, can allow for that creation in multiple ways. As perfect as the originating cast was (and it really was!), this play allows, in its spaces and nuances, for multiple varieties of interpretations, each of which will bring something to the creators and the viewers.

I spent some time after watching it trying to unpack why this little show—four actors and a marimba, a simple stage and simple lighting—had such an impact on me. I mean, I am a single, middle-aged man whose mother lives with him, and the show had a lot to say about that very specific relationship and who is taking care of whom, but it's much deeper than that obvious connection.

All of us have families, in all their messiness. The family in this play is messier than most, but we can all see some of ourselves in it. Rooted in the real life experiences of Clem, his brother Olivier, and their mother Catherine, this story rings deeply true.

(The Martini brothers have also penned a book about their experiences, more autobiographical than this play, with the rather on-the-nose title of *The Unravelling: How Our Caregiving Safety Net Came Unstrung and We Were Left Grasping at Threads, Struggling to Plait a New One,* as a follow-up to their award-winning—I know; I presented one of the awards!—*Bitter Medicine.*)

In *Cantata,* Dennis has been living with schizophrenia for decades. He's unable to work, but he has created a full life for himself, taking public transit to various programs and activities that build his community. It all works because he lives with his mother,

Irene, who keeps the train on the tracks, with occasional assists from her other son, Martin, who is juggling his own life, and work, and family commitments.

Irene is 89. She didn't sign up for this. Her family members are not that long-lived, and she certainly didn't expect to still be taking care of her son, who has been living with her for 40 years, at this point in her life. And she won't go to seniors' programs, with the terrible coffee and all the old people. (Okay, this part is a little too close to my life!)

But she's starting to forget things. She's starting to fail. And it's all about to fall apart.

It's almost cliché to point out that the aging of our population is the most important shift facing our society now and that we have to come up with a new way to manage our system of caregiving.

Caregiving. An interesting word, that. Towards the beginning of the play, Martin is asked if his mother takes care of Dennis. "They kind of look after each other," he responds. "I live close by and help out." For me, this simple line of dialogue was one of the most devastating, and the heart of what the story has to tell us.

What does it mean to give care, and to take care of one another? Do we do it out of love, or duty, or commitment, or because we have no other choice? What about those who are paid, or rather underpaid, to take on some of the burden? Why do they do it? Do they have no other choice?

Cantata doesn't try to provide the answers, nor does it make any grand pronouncements about What Should Be Done. It just tells the simple story of a little family, in all its deep complexity, and invites us all to reflect on what it means for every one of our families.

And yes, the ending is certainly not traditionally happy in any way, but it's real. It's about life. It's about how we all live our lives. And it's about resilience, the power to move forward, since that's really the only direction we have.

> — *Naheed K. Nenshi, 2023*
> *Naheed K. Nenshi is an avid theatre-goer.*
> *He served as Mayor of Calgary*
> *from 2010-2021.*

INTRODUCTION
CLEM MARTINI

I N 1977, my seventeen-year-old brother, Ben, began experiencing delusions and hallucinations. His personality rapidly changed, and in the summer following high school graduation he suddenly adopted an uncharacteristically aggressive manner. Following a violent incident, he was seized by police, taken to the psychiatric unit at the local hospital, and confined. After a period of several months, he was diagnosed as having schizophrenia, prescribed the psychotropic drug, Stelazine, and released back to my family, where he promptly purchased a gun and killed himself in the basement of our home. My family never fully recovered.

I'm well aware of the high stakes associated with family caregiving.

In 1982 my next oldest brother, Olivier, began experiencing similar delusions and hallucinations. He received disturbing messages from the television and passing cars telling him that he was a worthless loser and should kill himself. Eventually he took that advice and tried. I drove him to the hospital where he too was diagnosed as having schizophrenia. Like Ben, Olivier was prescribed Stelazine, and released to return home.

For over three decades Olivier shared a condominium with my mother—they grew close and helped one another out in so many ways—and my family built a network made up of family and friends, psychiatrists and psychiatric nurses, various psychiatric support groups, and of course, Olivier who contended each day with the side effects of the medication he took, the residual low-level paranoia he experienced, and the voices that continued to haunt him regardless of the amount or type of medication he took.

More than thirty years of survival judged by any metrics can be counted a success when it comes to schizophrenia, where the rate of suicide is so enormously high. (Twenty times higher than the general population according to the latest research published by the Centre for Addiction and Mental Health.) But what happens when the people in that network age, when the connective tissue begins to crumble and fall apart?

This play describes what can happen.

Our healthcare system relies on the many efforts of families offering assistance and sharing resources in this informal extended alliance, but the healthcare system fails to acknowledge the on-coming crisis as our population ages. It's not just one family that is aging and wondering how to proceed, but hundreds of thousands of families facing a similar predicament.

It was my mother's desire that she age in place, and for the longest time—until the wheels came off that particular car—my family attempted to ensure that both Olivier and my mother received care in the apartment they had lived in for decades. I enrolled in several international online courses regarding caregiving for those with dementia, as well as those suffering psychosis, hoping that I would be better equipped to help. I recall attending a chat room in one of the courses and receiving a message from a participant who wrote that she was in her eighties, had terminal cancer, and didn't know what arrangements she could take for her adult son who suffered from a mental illness and had lived most of his life with her. "Who will care for him now?" she asked. "Does anyone have any advice?" Another participant expressed a different perspective. He had coped with a severe mental illness as best he could for most of his life by living with his supportive parents, but his parents were now old and frail. How could he possibly care for them, he wondered, and what was he to do when they died?

There's a hard truth that contextualizes family caregiving, and that is that the options are limited. Back in the sixties and seventies protests were launched against the institutionalized care that had been provided for those diagnosed with mental illness. The large psychiatric asylums that had provided 'treatment' for those with mental illnesses for decades proved to be ineffective at best, and dangerous at worst. Neglect, and abuse, both physical and sexual, were found to be systemic. By the eighties, asylums had been shuttered, and the majority of long-term psychiatric beds at hospitals, closed. The considerable government funding that had gone into maintaining these facilities was supposed to flow into smaller community facilities that would assist with socialization and treatment. Instead, when the institutions were shuttered, the funds disappeared as well. For those coping with mental illnesses there were few places to receive care, and prison and homelessness became very real potential outcomes. Today, prisons are the number one caregiver for those with severe mental illnesses. It's not uncommon for individuals to receive their first diagnosis of a mental illness in jail, and their first treatment. The homeless shelters of this country are all oversubscribed by those struggling with mental illnesses.

Those suffering from dementia—one of the most prevalent mental disorders—are also some of the worst served, their care being systemically, chronically, underfunded and under supported. Because they are elderly, because they are viewed as being at the end of term and perhaps 'beyond saving', because society finds them embarrassing, the resources provided for their care are particularly insufficient. Reports have been issued time and again (The Royal Society sponsored report, 2020, The Organization for Health Action's report, 2020, The Public Health Agency's report, 2019) indicating that care for the aged is miserably resourced. The Covid pandemic exposed just how poorly those with dementia have been cared for, and so many paid for this tightfistedness with their lives.

Providing care within a family may be the better option, but it's not easy. There's little medical support, little coordinated communication between health services, and unlike hospitals or asylums where when staff retires someone new is hired, the family caregiving model rarely has a transition plan.

I wrote *Cantata* as a way of raising awareness and reaching out to those that I know are struggling. I have intentionally written *Cantata* to be produced in a spare, economic, bare-bones manner. It requires little to be staged beyond space, lights, actors, a marimba, and determination. It can be staged, literally, anywhere.

When *Cantata: Rumours of My Crazy, Useless Life* was first produced by Sage Theatre, I attended nearly every performance. It was mounted in a small blackbox theater, with the marimba positioned maybe fifteen feet from the front row seats. The actors performed even closer—the experience was intended to be intimate. Seats sold well and houses were full, but it was apparent from the outset that we were drawing a different crowd: a raw, emotionally invested audience. People were frequently moved to an extent that they had to remain behind after the show ended to gather themselves. Audiences held hands during the show. Many people wept. Every night that I attended, once the curtain dropped, individuals sought me out to say, 'That story is our story too. We felt overwhelmed as well. We didn't know where to turn. We couldn't talk about it with anyone. That happened to us.'

This play is dedicated to all those who are out there, coping as best they can, trying to care for loved ones, improvising solutions for the new challenges that emerge every day, feeling underqualified, facing judgment when they fail, on the phone to various over-subscribed government help lines where they are inevitably put on hold, or told to leave a message and then never receive a response. I see you. I wrote this play based upon my family's experience, not because I think my family is special, but because I know we're not.

—*Clem Martini, 2023*

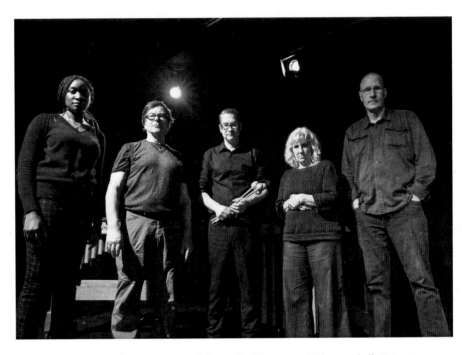

L to R: Precious Akpoguma, Duval Lang, Rod Squance, Val Campbell, Brian Jenson

Photos throughout: Cliff Kirschhoff

CAST

Premiere Production
Sage Theatre at C-Space
Calgary, Alberta, Canada

DUVAL LANG— Martin Berenger
BRIAN JENSON— Dennis Berenger
VAL CAMPBELL— Irene Berenger
PRECIOUS AKPOGUMA— Psychiatrist/Counsellor/
Bank Manager/Nurse, Growling Patient

JASON MEHMEL— Director
ROD SQUANCE— Compose/Marimba player
EMILY PARKHOUSE— Stage Manager
CALUM MAUNIER— Designer

Workshop and Staged Reading
Sage Theatre at C-Space
Calgary, Alberta, Canada

VAL PEARSON— Irene Berenger
MIKE TAN— Dennis Berenger
LOUISE CASEMORE— Martin Berenger
JANELLE COOPER— Psychiatrist/Counsellor/
Bank Manager/Nurse, Growling Patient

JASON MEHMEL— Director
ROD SQUANCE— Composer/Marimba player

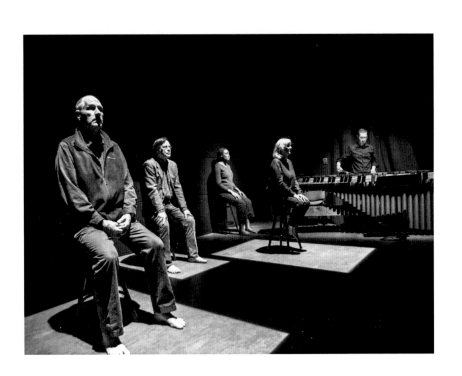

CANTATA
RUMOURS OF MY CRAZY, USELESS LIFE

CLEM MARTINI

All sounds, voices, and music are produced by four actors and a marimba. Actors will adopt and shed other minor characters as necessary.

Time is fractured.

Cast

Irene Berenger: elderly, the mother of Martin and Dennis
Martin Berenger: the younger son
Dennis Berenger: the older son
Psychiatrist/Counsellor/Bank Manager
Nurse, Growling Patient

The actors are barefoot.
Their costumes reflect a simple, spare look.

Setting

The setting consists of three tall stools, and a marimba, on an otherwise bare stage. The stools are employed as the action requires, becoming car seats, hospital beds, walkers.

The marimba is fluent, at times expressing a score for movements on stage, other times articulating an activity—an elevator door opening, time passing, snowfall—and other times responding to a line of dialogue as though it was a character itself.

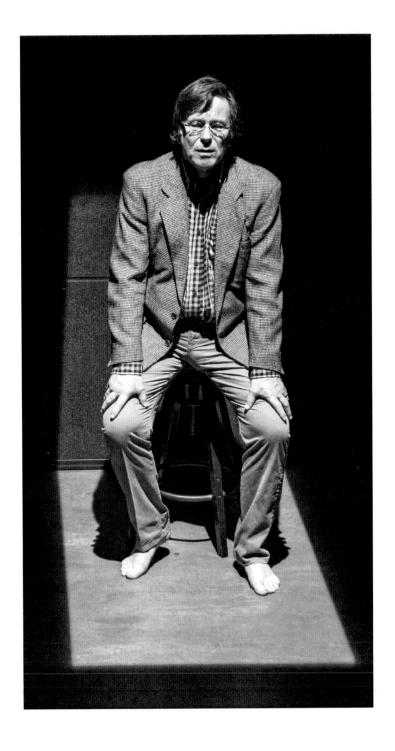

CANTATA
RUMOURS OF MY CRAZY, USELESS LIFE

Act One

Darkness.

A faint, slight trill of the marimba is heard, ghostly, followed by the quick sound of something shaking...a rattlesnake? A maraca? A beat, then, still.

In darkness, the cast draws an extended intake of breath for a count of eight, then releases that breath in an abrupt puff.

Pause.

That cycle is repeated.

Pause.

It is repeated again.

Lights rise on Martin.

Another breath by the actors, and Martin launches—

Martin   It's early and dark when the telephone rings.

(The marimba indicates a phone.)

I haven't had breakfast yet and am just set up at the dining room table looking over some notes.

(Lights rise on Irene as well.)

Irene   Something is definitely wrong, I can't make any sense of him.

(*Lights rise on Dennis and the Psychiatrist as well.*)

Psychiatrist   (*Speaking as she types an email*) I'm blown away that he's been discharged without the unit first consulting me. I guess they at least had the courtesy of faxing me the discharge summary.

Irene   He's been like that since he was released from the hospital the other day.

Martin   Can you hear me?

Dennis, can you hear me?

Dennis   (*Slowly, deciphering what he sees*)
There are words.
I can tell there are words.
But it is like I'm encased in Jell-O.

Psychiatrist   (*As before*) He missed his last appointment, so I called him. He was clearly not himself. Unfortunately, I am out of the country for the next three weeks, starting tomorrow.

Irene   He stares off into space, doesn't respond when I talk to him.

Dennis   The words appear, just outside the Jell-O, as bubbles I can't touch and don't appear to have meaning.

Martin   Dennis?

Dennis   And it's strange.
I don't know how long I have been this way
And I don't know how long it will last, or if it will ever end.

Psychiatrist   (*As before*) I will check my email daily, though, so we can try to manage this and I will see him on my first day back. Worst case scenario, if he continues to decline please take him to ER and ask for a psychiatric hospital admission, and we'll try to sort this out.

Martin   Dennis, can you follow me? I'm taking you to emergency. Can you follow me?

Dennis   Yes.

(*The musician begins playing the marimba, a quick melody.*)

Irene   Hello?
Hello?
Hello. I've tried calling three times today and I can't get hold of anyone. Is there anyone that can talk to—

Martin   Mom.

Irene   Hello? Is this the machine—

Martin   Mom, it's me.

Irene   Is it you? It's not the machine?

Martin   It's me.

Irene   Well. Finally!
I've tried calling ALL DAY—(*the following conversation overlaps, as many of their future conversations will overlap.*)—and zilch—

Martin   You called at 2:00—

Irene   —all I get is the answering machine—

Martin   —2:00 and then at 2:15, 2:25, 2:35—

Irene   —I get so *lonely* sitting here—

Martin   —3:15—

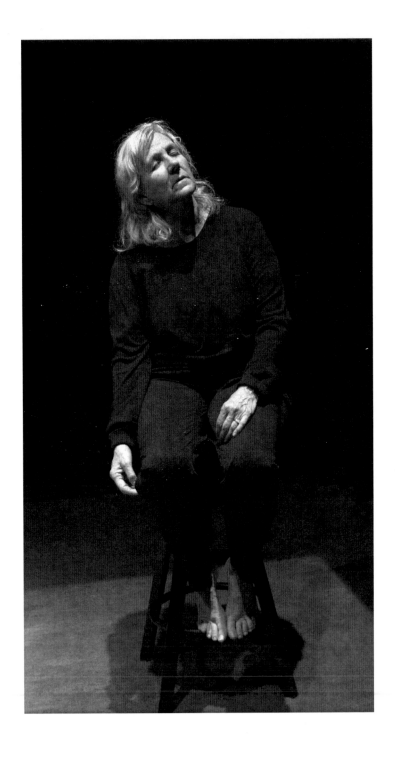

Irene	—with Dennis gone,
Martin	—I know it's tough with him in the hospital—
Irene	—and *who knows* when he'll get out—
Martin	—Dr. Best thinks he's stabilized and will be released soon,
Irene	—'soon', what does that mean—
Martin	—and in the meantime—
Irene	—it could mean days, weeks—
Martin	—you could attend some of those senior events we've suggested—
Irene	—Agh, I don't want to go somewhere with *old* people and *play games*, I'm too old for board games—
Martin	—It's about socializing with people your age. Just try them—
Irene	—and the coffee is *terrible*—
Martin	—bring your own coffee—
Irene	—I want to see some of my family—is it asking too much to want talk to my sons?
Martin	It is if I'm at work and not at home, so can't answer the phone. You know the hours, why would you call me when you know I'm at work?
Irene	Why can't *you* take me to those seniors events?—
Martin	—Because I'm *at work*, that's why I wasn't home when you called—
Irene	—You're always at work, I don't know when to call—

Martin	—I work the *same* hours every day. It's pointless calling me during work hours, call me when I'm at home.
Irene	You're never home!
Martin	That's not true.
Irene	You're never home!
Martin	I'm home now. You're talking to me!
	(*Beat*)
	I'll come over.
	(*He hangs up.*)
Irene	(*A different tone, she confides with the audience*) I forgot he was at work.

(*Marimba plays softly underneath.*)

Life plays bitter tricks and you're not always able to do what you want. I never expected to live to eighty-nine, I never expected to live to *seventy*. My mother died when she was thirty-three, my father, sixty-six, my grandparents were gone before I was born.

A month ago I lost my keys. Thought I lost them. I didn't *really* lose them, they appeared later deep in my inner coat pocket, it extends further into the liner than I realized, but at the time I *thought* I'd lost them so could not get into the apartment. It was a disaster. My mind isn't as sharp as it once was.

I'd returned from a special service at the Unitarian Church. Dennis was attending one of his psychiatric support groups and wouldn't return home till late, so there was no chance that he could unlock the door.

Another resident was going up in the elevator from the parkade, and they were able to let me upstairs, but then I had to wait, sitting on the top stairs, for about five hours, until Dennis arrived. Waiting. Waiting. You spend a lot of your time waiting when you get old.

That's what I'm saying. You are not always able to do what you want.

It is not possible to do things the way you would like them. It's not possible to do some things at all. But it isn't worth making a fuss.

Life carries on. It carries on and I have learned not to get upset just because everything doesn't go the way I planned.

Martin   At seven a.m. I drive to Mom and Dennis's place, unlock the door, let myself in. The apartment is dark. At first I think that she must still be in bed, then I see a little light spilling from the open washroom door.

Mom? I call to warn her that I've entered the apartment.

It's a challenge to determine how loud to pitch my voice. Her hearing is poor at the best of times, even with her hearing aids in, and she frequently doesn't install them until after her first cup of coffee. If I'm too quiet, she won't hear. If I'm too loud she'll startle and take a fall.

Mom? I call again, a bit louder. Nothing. I close the door to the hallway and move toward the bathroom where I find my mother staring at herself in the mirror. She's naked, so I step back.

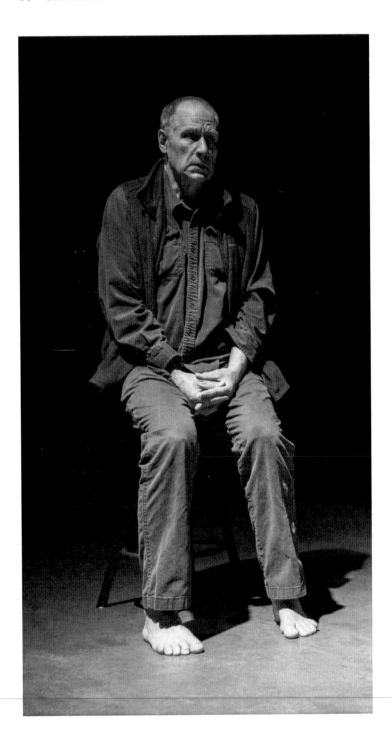

	Hello, I say, louder than before, hoping to get her attention.
	Mom, are you okay?
Irene	No.
Martin	I step into the room. She is leaning forward, gripping the lip of the sink, studying her reflection.
Irene	Something's wrong.
Martin	What is?
Irene	I don't know.
Martin	Is this everything you came with?
Dennis	Yes.
Martin	And they've signed you out?
Dennis	Yes.
Martin	And you feel good?
Dennis	Yes.
Martin	Your meds are all in order?
	(*Dennis shakes his pill container*)
Martin	Okay, let's go.
	How was last night?
Dennis	There was a lot of drama.
Martin	What happened?
Dennis	One guy on the unit beat his head against the wall. Blood everywhere. He was restrained. Then a biker was admitted, big, bearded, tattooed, shouting, f this and f that, and they couldn't get him to sit down, I'm not f-ing sitting down, I'm not f-ing sitting down, the police came, I guess he was involved in some

	kind of prior crime. They cuffed him and escorted him out.
Martin	That's a lot of drama.
Dennis	Yea. Too much drama. I didn't think I'd end up spending my sixtieth birthday in the psych ward. I'm glad I'm out of there.
Martin	Me too. Here's my car.
Oliver	Hope I never go back.
Martin	Amen. Do up your seat belt.
	(The car starts.)
	So.
Dennis	Yea?
Martin	You've noticed that Mom's been forgetting things?
Dennis	Sometimes. Yea?
Martin	Things are changing.
Dennis	What things?
Martin	The counsellor is a middle-aged woman with flushed cheeks and air of constantly being slightly out of breath and behind in her schedule. Her office is compact—
Counsellor	—Sit down—
Martin	—barely able to accommodate her desk and lamp
Counsellor	—just push that aside on the desk—
Martin	—and I wonder what this room might have been when it was originally part of an elementary school—the broom closet maybe?

Counsellor	What brought you here?
Martin	My mother has been declining for several years, she's had a number of falls, and I called Health Link and they said I should meet with—
Counsellor	—Over what period of time?
Martin	Declining? A couple of years—three years? More recently incidents have happened with greater frequency—
Counsellor	—how mobile is she?
Martin	She can get by with the help of a cane although her doctor has urged her to use her walker—
Counsellor	Does she live alone?
Martin	My older brother lives with her. He has schizophrenia.
Counsellor	Does she look after him?
Martin	They kind of look after each other. I live close by and help out—
Counsellor	Does she drive?
Martin	Unfortunately.
Counsellor	Ha.
Martin	Terrible driver.
Counsellor	So many of them are.
Martin	She'll kill herself.
Counsellor	Or someone else. (*Thrusts a paper at him*) Write your address here. I'll have material sent to you.

Martin	When she doesn't use her walker she falls, and she's beginning to show signs of dementia, forgetfulness, irritability, she phones all the time, forgets that I'm at work—
Counsellor	So common.
Martin	—then forgets that we spoke—
Counsellor	—You'll need these as well—
Martin	—she was standing in the washroom the other day, naked, staring in the mirror, kept saying something's wrong, something's wrong, I don't know what it was—
Counsellor	—Terrible—
Martin	She was pretty upset.
Counsellor	Read these. How old is your mother and how frail?
Martin	Approaching ninety—
Counsellor	And take this.
Martin	—and pretty frail. She's broken bones falling, wrist, feet, nose—
Counsellor	It's essential that you have her assessed for her mental and physical competencies.
Martin	This is the first that I hear of an assessment. I will learn that the assessments never end.
Counsellor	The assessment will provide the medical authorities—
Martin	Never. A chain of perpetual, ongoing, never-ending assessments.
Counsellor	—with the information necessary to decide what level of care is most appropriate: care in home or placement in an assisted living

facility. Don't waste any time. It can take months to years,

Martin   Really?

Counsellor   Months to years to get into an assisted living facility. So if there is the remotest chance that this will become an eventuality, you should begin making your preparations immediately. (*Staring at him*) Immediately.

(Dennis delivers a quick shake of a pill container, like a maraca.)

Dennis   She's up every morning early, calls me.

Irene   Dennis!

Dennis   Gets coffee ready. Makes sure I take my meds.

(Delivers another quick shake of the pill container, then pours pills into his hand and swallows them.)

Now, after coffee I head off to my group sessions and art classes. Circle of Friends. Schizophrenia Society. Creative Living. Peer Options. But I remember when there wasn't any of that. When there was no one. No organizations. No support groups. When I was first diagnosed, it was survive the best you could on your own. Deal with the drugs' side effects on your own. Deal with the delusions on your own. I would lie in bed for hours, sweating, too depressed to get up, too afraid to lift the sheets, then she'd call me. Force me to climb out of bed. Make me breakfast, then make me eat it. Maybe take me out for a drive. Sometimes she'd pack a picnic and we'd go out to the mountains and sit under pine trees by a river.

It's almost forty years that I've lived with her.

(Phone rings)

Dennis	Can you come over?
Martin	Why what's up?
Dennis	The phone's not working.
Martin	Where are you?
Dennis	I'm calling from the neighbour's line.
Martin	I arrive—Hi—Dennis is sunk into the couch looking defeated, my mother stares out the window, I pick up the phone. Was the phone dropped?
Dennis	No.
Martin	There's no dial tone.
Dennis	No.
Martin	I follow the cord to the wall. Okay, the phone's plugged in. How long has it been like this?
Dennis	Today.
Martin	Is the phone bill paid?
Dennis	I don't know.
Martin	Mom?
Irene	What?
Martin	Is the phone bill paid?
Irene	I don't know.
Martin	Well, how have the bills been paid in the past?

	(*Beat*)
	Who pays the bills?
Dennis	Mom.
Martin	Where are the bills kept?
Irene	In my purse.
Martin	In your purse? Can I have a look? I reach in and at the bottom of the deep leather pocket there they are, dozens and dozens, and they're all, every one of them, unopened.

(*To Liv*) These are unopened. (*To Mom*) Why haven't you opened them? This is a final notice, and this is a notice to disconnect.

And this one.

Gas, electric, cable TV—they're all in arrears. Why have you put them in your purse unopened?

Mom, why have you put them in your purse unopened?

(*Beat*)

Okay. First, I'm going to get the phone working, and then I'm going to get all your bills arranged to be debited automatically. Do you understand?

I make an appointment to meet with her bank manager. When I pick her up she's seated, her coat buttoned up. Have you got your driver's license?

Irene	Yes.
Martin	And your banking card?
Irene	Everything I need is in this purse—

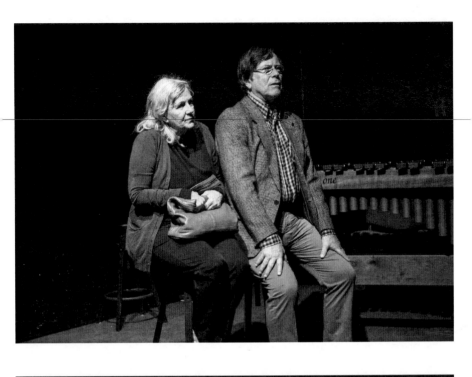

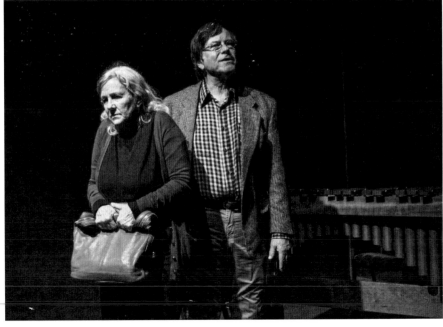

Martin	Okay then—
Irene	—my whole life is in here! When you get to my age, it pays to have everything handy. I don't want to be running somewhere to fetch my cheque book, or my health card, or banking card, social insurance number, or a pen, or nail clippers, or hairbrush, or pencil, or paper. You run a little slower when you get to be my age.
Martin	Okay. You've got everything. Let's go.

I help her to the car.

But as I place the car in gear and drive out I notice something. While waiting in the bank lobby to meet the manager I begin to detect an odour. And the longer we wait the more convinced I become that it's coming from my mother—and that everyone in the bank can detect it as well. And they all know that it's coming from us.

I start to sweat.

The receptionist approaches, glances at my mother, frowns briefly, then guides us through a hallway to an office, where we squeeze into tiny seats at the manager's majestic desk.

The bank manager stiffly guides us through the procedure involved with my taking over her financial affairs. As he speaks, I hear the words, but I'm not paying attention. I feel myself slowly melting. I take the form from him, tell him my mother and I will fill it out, shake his hand, and my mother and

I leave, but as we exit the bank I realize that there is a very special currency that is issued when you deal with dementia and it's issued in varying denominations of shame. My mother, too embarrassed to warn me, receives her payment. I, too embarrassed to cancel the meeting, receive mine.

We drive back. My suggestion that we stop at the grocery store and purchase a couple of new packages of Depends is greeted by my mother with silence as she turns to stare out the passenger side window.

Dennis	I was walking home from the c-train when I noticed a car slowly following me. As I stopped at an intersection I looked through the car's window and saw a man pressing his face against the glass, making a face at me, sticking his finger up his nose, and I realized he's laughing at me. Poking his friend, pointing me out, daring me to fight and I am resolved from now on to carry a tire iron with me in case that car, or any car, or any man in a car, or that particular son of a bitch follows me again, I will pull out that tire iron. I will pull it out and I will use it! I just want to make him think I think I think I think!
Irene	(*Calling from her bed*) Can you help me?
Martin	What?
Irene	Can you. Help. Me. Up?
Martin	Where's your walker?
Irene	I don't know.

Martin	How did you even get to bed without it?
	(*Seeing it*)
	Here it is.
	And where are your—
Irene	I have to go to the washroom!
Martin	—dentures? Okay, let's stand you up.
	Where are your dentures?
Irene	What?
Martin	Your *dentures*? Teeth? Where are they?
Irene	Stolen.
Martin	What?
	(*She slips into the washroom.*)
	Did you say 'stolen'?
	I look about the apartment.
	Her dentures must be somewhere—how many places can you put dentures?
	She reappears.
	Who stole your dentures?
Irene	The plumber.
Martin	The plumber?
Irene	Yes.
Martin	The plumber stole your dentures?
Irene	He came to look at the sink yesterday—it's plugged again—I put my dentures in a glass of water in the washroom and he took them.
Martin	You saw him take them?
Irene	Yes.
Martin	You *saw him* take them?

Irene	They were there when he arrived and weren't when he was gone.
Martin	Why would he want your old dentures?
Irene	I don't know.
Martin	That seems unlikely.
Irene	That's the way some people are. Old people don't count, so they take their dentures.
Martin	We embark on a time of The Great Losing. Over a stretch of several weeks she loses her dentures, her watch—
Irene	It was here earlier.
Martin	—her wallet, her glasses, her hearing aids, her watch—
Irene	It was on my wrist. Right there.
Martin	—her dentures, her driver's licence— hurray! —her glasses, her *dentures*—God! Just take them out the same time each night and put them in the case! I leave a message with Home Care asking that they send help for my mother.
	I broach the subject of moving to assisted living with my mother.
Irene	Noooo. There's no point moving anywhere *at my age*.
Martin	Wouldn't you like to live somewhere where your needs were taken care of, someplace new—
Irene	Noooo. Why would I move someplace new *at my age*? I've lived here since we sold the old home. I'm familiar with everything. Yes,

	it's difficult to get about, but that's the thing about growing old—
Martin & Irene	—It's not for the weak.
Martin	Then I arrive one afternoon. Dennis has settled into his usual place enveloped by the couch, half asleep.
	You look tired.
Dennis	She fell again last night.
Martin	When?
Dennis	Around three. Got out of bed and found her crying on the floor.
Martin	Where did she go down?
Dennis	By the rocking chair. Give me a hand up.
Martin	Your back hurt?
Dennis	I did something to it—Ow—when I lifted her. She couldn't get—Ow—up. I should have learned something practical in school.
Martin	Like what?
Dennis	How to lift someone from the floor.
Martin	I don't think they offer lessons in that.
Dennis	No, the only thing that they cared about at school was discipline, but only discipline for the weak. Bullies were left to their own devices.
	Although school did prepare me for the Hell that is the work world.
Martin	(*Grunts his displeasure*)

Dennis	For years I worked with a cabal called the Training Centre—
Martin	—Don't start—
Dennis	—and the only thing they were ever interested in was breaking me—
Martin	—No one there was trying to break you.
Dennis	Of course they were.
Martin	Why would anyone 'try to break you'?
Dennis	So that I would be prepared to accept my role as a labour slave.
Martin	You know when you talk like that you sound—
Dennis	What? Crazy?
Martin	Irrational.
Dennis	For years I worked as a security guard in the most miserable places on Earth abandoned factories, and isolated, crumbling construction sites, until the loneliness nearly killed me, then they were happy.
Martin	Who?
Dennis	Them.
Martin	Who was happy?
Dennis	All of them—
Martin	—Ah!—
Dennis	—And *then* after I ended up in the psych ward they sent me for retraining so I could fit in but by that time I was too broken, and they put me on disability.
Martin	That's absurd too.
Dennis	Every absurd thing I say—

Martin	—Why frame everything in the most negative possible way—
Dennis	—I could match with three of yours—
Martin	—All I'm saying—
Dennis	—You don't know. You don't.
Martin	Home Care, returns my call. They tell me they will send someone over for, what else…
	(*Doorbell rings.*)
Homecare	Hello?
Martin	…An assessment.
Homecare	I'm Karen from Homecare and I've come by to have a conversation with your mother.
Irene	Karen *who*? From *what*?
Martin	Homecare.
	I watch the Homecare Staff taking everything in as she enters—
Irene	*What?*
Martin & Dennis	*Homecare!*
Martin	—the poor condition of the apartment, the adult son, my mother, and I see her stiffen.
Homecare	I enter the apartment and immediately smell the powerfully unpleasant odour of urine. I introduce myself and try to make the old woman feel at ease.
Martin	She slaps on an artificial smile, and adopts a tone that you would take with a small child.
Homecare	Hello, I'll be asking you a few questions, there are no wrong answers.

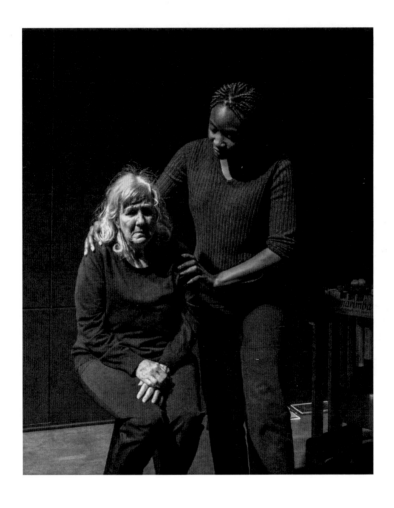

Irene	Why is she talking like that?
Homecare	Can you cook for yourself?—
Irene	*What?* (*To Martin*) She's mumbling, I can't hear her—
Martin	She begins over-articulating every word she says and shifts and positions herself directly in front of my mother—
Homecare	Is this better?
Martin	—too close. My mother bristles.
Homecare	—she doesn't hear and frowns at me like an angry bear—what a terrible old woman —I move closer so she can hear me. She raises her eyebrows as though I have done something incredibly rude. (*Over-articulating each syllable*) Can You Cook for Yourself?
Irene	Can I *cook* for myself? Do I look like an idiot?
Homecare	She objects to everything I say—
Irene	Of course I can cook for myself.
Homecare	And *repeats* everything I say.
Irene	Can I cook for myself? I've been cooking since I was old enough to reach the burner on the stovetop. I have been cooking since I was eight. Since my mother died.
Homecare	Are you able to look after yourself? Dress yourself, feed yourself—
Irene	What?
Martin	She's asking if you can dress yourself—
Irene	Dress myself??
Homecare	What I'm trying to determine—

Irene	—What a load of nonsense!
Homecare	—is your level of need.
Irene	Dress myself??
Homecare	Are you able to *look* after yourself?
Irene	Who are *you*? Of course I can *look* after myself. I have been *looking* after myself for over *eighty-eight* years. I have been *looking after* myself since before you were born.
Homecare	Can you clean yourself?
Irene	What?
Martin	She asked if you can clean yourself.
Irene	Did you say *clean yourself*?
Homecare	Can you? (*to Martin*) Can she? Wash? Bathe yourself?
Martin	Not really.
Irene	I clean myself very well, thank you.
Homecare	Do you pee frequently?
Irene	Do I *pee*? Did she say 'do I pee?'
Martin	Mom.
Homecare	Can you clean yourself after you pee?
Irene	Can I clean myself after? Do you—
Homecare	Can you wipe yourself—
Irene	—Do you think I'm a baby?—
Homecare	—I don't think you're a baby—
Irene	— Do you think I'm an infant? Do you think that I'm stupid?
Homecare	I don't think you're stupid.
Irene	She thinks I'm stupid.

Martin	She doesn't think you're stupid.
Homecare	I don't think you're stupid.
Martin	Nobody thinks you're stupid.
Homecare	Nothing like that.
	(*to the audience*) She will need much, *much* more help than we can provide, but I initiate what we can offer.
	(*to Martin*) We will send a person three mornings a week, as a pilot. That person will support her with showering, dressing, and provide some light tidying up.
Martin	Homecare commences.
Homecare 2	Good Morning.
Irene	Who are *you*?
Martin	And is an immediate disaster.
	They send a young man to our mother's door, who announces—
Homecare 2	I've come to administer your shower.
Irene	*You*?? Come again —*You* shower *me*!!
Martin	Mom responds with fury—
Irene	I'll show *you* showering!
Homecare 2	Take it easy.
Irene	Aah!
	(*She chases him around and between the stools, remarkably quickly given that she is employing a walker.*)
Homecare 2	Whoa! Lady! Lady!
Martin	—chasing him out into the hallway—
Homecare 2	—Whoa!—

Martin	—shouting as he goes—
Irene	And don't *ever* come back!
Martin	And then she phones me—
Irene	Did *you* mistakenly believe I wanted to be scrubbed by a *boy*??
Martin	And if this was the kind of help she could expect—
Irene	You can cancel it all right away—
Martin	I call Homecare and they apologize—
Homecare	No, it was not our intention to offend, it was a miscommunication—
Irene	No, no, no, I don't want anything to do with them! Nothing!
Martin	—and assure us it was all a mistake—
Homecare	—just a terrible, terrible miscommunication—
Irene	—Nothing!—
Martin	—and would be corrected. But it's too late.
Irene	I don't need it, and I don't want it!
	I don't want it, I don't want it, I don't want it!
Martin	But then three weeks later.
Irene	Martin, help!
Martin	The phone rings. It's mid-afternoon.
	Mom? What is it?
Irene	Help!
Martin	Where are you?
Irene	At home! I've fallen.
Martin	Isn't there anyone with you

Irene	No, Dennis is at his programs. I've been lying on the floor for hours.
Martin	What about Homecare—
Irene	I sent them all away—after I fell I dragged myself over to the—
Martin	To the what?
Irene	To the—
Martin	The door, the bed?
Irene	—the coffee table and knocked over the phone with my cane. Help, help, help!
Martin	Are you bleeding?
Irene	No.
Martin	Have you broken anything? Should I call an ambulance?
Irene	No, no, no! I just can't get up, I can't pull myself up! And my hip—Help, help!—
Martin	Mom! I'm going to call parameds for you!
Irene	I don't *want them*! I don't want them!
Martin	All right.
Irene	Just come as quick as you can, Martin! Just come.
Martin	It'll take me at least twenty minutes from the office.

I send a note cancelling my grad class and climb into my car.

She's lying on the floor when I arrive, an angry red lump rising from her forehead, blood trickling from a nostril. Her great wooden chair that she normally sits in and surveys the world from, is sprawled over on its side.

Mom?

Irene	At last, at last.
Martin	What happened?
Irene	I was walking from the kitchen to the chair and then—down.
Martin	Is anything sprained or broken?
Irene	No.
Martin	Are you hurt anywhere?
Irene	No.
Martin	You're sure?
Irene	Yes, I just can't get up, and my hip.... Put the chair back in its place, and set me up in it.
Martin	Okay—

(*He considers how exactly he will lift her.*)

I'll take you around the shoulders.

(*He does so, lifts and she releases a long sustained, full-throated, scream*)

Irene	*Aaaahh!*
Martin	Mom!
Irene	*Aaaaah!*

(*It's deafening*)

Martin	What's wrong? What's wrong, should I set you back down? Is something broken?
Irene	No!

Put me in the chair, put me in the chair, put me in the chair,

Aaaaaah!

(*She is placed in the chair. She immediately calms.*)

Ah.

(*Total Silence. Beat*)

Martin	Are you all right?
Dennis	A woman in Transylvania had a mental illness.
Irene	I'm fine.
Dennis	The Nuns felt she was possessed, so she was chained to a cross by her priest, starved and beaten for days and—
Martin	Where did you read this?
Dennis	—exorcised—they reported it on television —and eventually killed. The priest gave the boot to the devil. Wouldn't that be better?
Martin	Better than what?
Dennis	Than this.
Martin	What are you talking about?
Dennis	Wouldn't it be better if everyone with a mental illness was burned at the stake?
Martin	—Agh—
Dennis	—Isn't that what the public wants?
Martin	Don't be ridiculous.
Dennis	It's not ridiculous.
Martin	When has anyone ever said—
Dennis	They don't have to say it—
Martin	—they wanted to burn you at the stake?
Dennis	—they *think* it.

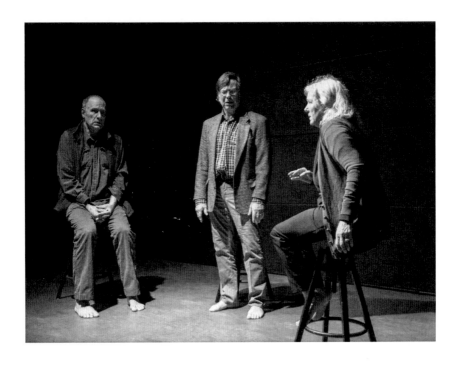

Martin	Nobody thinks that.
Dennis	The government just announced that they are cutting the Assured Income for the Severely Disabled. Again. They withdrew funding to our support groups. Again. Our occupational therapist was fired. Our writing class was cancelled. No money. Every time the government needs to find savings, the first thing they do is stick it to the crazies. It's death by a thousand hits and the only place I fit in in this society is begging. Or burning.
Martin	What's the point of saying something like that?
Dennis	I'm telling it the way it is.
Martin	That's just pointlessly negative.
Dennis	It only seems that way to you because you don't understand.
Martin	Dennis and I convene a meeting. I pull two chairs in from the dining room, Dennis takes his place on the sofa. Mom sits as usual in her high-backed wooden chair. I outline the situation.
Irene	Dennis, have you taken your pills?
Dennis	Yes.
Irene	Have you?
Dennis	I said *yes!*
Martin	Okay. Mom, we need to talk. Your health is worsening, your hygiene is a problem—
Irene	I don't have a problem with hygiene— (*Martin continues over top*)

Martin	—*and* the apartment is falling apart. You need to accept more help, you *need* someone to come in, clean up and prepare meals.
Irene	I don't want anyone *fussing* around me and getting in the way—
Martin	Your legs have become swollen and infected. You *need* someone to administer your medication.
Irene	I take my medication.
Martin	But not in the order or the amount that's required.
Irene	The pharmacy won't give it to me in a clear manner—
Martin	—They give it to you in marked blister packs—
Irene	—I hate those blister packs!
Martin	—they're marked each day of the week—
Irene	—Those blister packs are a confusing, gawdawful, unholy mess, all the pills *clumped* together—
Martin	—you took the first *week's* worth in one day.
Irene	I did not.
Martin	You did.
Irene	Someone *meddled* with it—
Martin	—Nobody meddled with it—
Irene	—maybe those teenagers from Homecare meddled—
Martin	—They aren't teenagers—
Irene	—they're worse than teenagers—
Martin	—how are they *worse* than teenagers? What

does that even mean? And nobody meddled. You remind Dennis to take his medication, and *you* need someone to remind you, and you need someone to help you shower.

Irene   Come again, I don't need a child to shower me. I have cleaned myself my whole life—

Martin   —The apartment smells, Mom—

Irene   —when I was in the army I learned how to clean myself with a sponge.

Martin   —*You* smell.—

Irene   —If you do it right it can give you a complete and thorough cleaning.

Martin   But you *can't.* That's why you need Homecare's help.

Irene   *Help*? They are the opposite of helpful. They are just teenagers—

Martin   —I'm telling you they're not teenagers!—

Irene   Exactly! They're worse than teenagers—

Martin   —Will you stop.—

Irene   —they don't know how to do a single thing.—

Martin   —Just stop—

Irene   —How to sweep, how to boil water.

Martin   They're in their twenties, minimum, they're legally not permitted to hire anyone less than eighteen—

Irene   —They haven't learned *anything*—

Martin   —and everyone knows how to boil water, who doesn't know how to boil water?—

Irene	—They don't know how to make a bed, if they make it I just have to strip it and make it all up again. If they wipe the counter they just brush the crumbs on the floor. They fiddle, fiddle, fiddle, fiddle and create more problems than they fix. I'll tell you what they are, they are Home Care*less*.
	(*Phone rings*)
Martin	Hello?
Homecare	Yes, Mr. Berenger?
Martin	Yes.
Homecare	I'm calling from Homecare. Do you remember me?
Martin	I remember you.
Homecare	We've been attempting to provide support for your Mother.
Martin	Yes, and I appreciate it.
Homecare	The report I have received is troubling.
Martin	I imagine she's difficult.
Homecare	Our records show that she has refused showering assistance nine out of ten times in the last three weeks. She has declined any help with cleaning or helping about the house.
Martin	My brother says she allowed them to put some dishes away, dust, get her some water—
Homecare	—She won't permit any assistance in helping her out of her bed, or even in making the bed.
Martin	She's stubborn.
Homecare	Yes, well, I'm calling to say that we are cancelling our services as of this week.

Martin	Really? Cancelling them?
Homecare	We have to be realistic.
Martin	Isn't there something we can change or adjust?
Homecare	We can't pay people to show up and do nothing.
	She needs more than we can offer.
Martin	Homecare ceases visitation, and the small things they could do, come to a halt. My mother develops ulcers that then become infected. We try to support her but she falls, and then falls again.
Dennis	Today I was chased off the c-train.
Martin	Nothing we say makes a difference.
Dennis	A drunk sat across the aisle, cursing no one in particular. Then his attention shifted to me—
Drunk	Look at you. Look at *you*.
Dennis	—It's not the first time that kind of thing has happened. Drunks can sense the weakest link. I got up and moved to the end of the car to avoid trouble,
Drunk	—Where do you think *you're* going?
Dennis	—but he followed me, muttering—
Drunk	—fucktard—
Dennis	—I got off the train, he followed me out—
Drunk	—Fucking retarded fucktard—
Dennis	—I walked faster. He sped up till he was right behind me, talking louder—
Drunk	—Freak! You're a freak!—

Dennis	— pushing me in the back, shouting in my ear—
Drunk	—You want a piece of me!—
Dennis	—Pushing me! I ran into a Safeway.—
Drunk	—*You want a piece of me!*—
Dennis	—While he pressed flat against the glass window shouting—
Drunk	—I'll *kick* your weiny ass!!—
Dennis	That kind of stuff happens allll the time.

I try to stay active. I walked to the writing group to enter my written piece for the Canadian Mental Health Association's monthly newsletter into the computer — but it will never get published because the story is based on the Decameron which is an ancient Italian book written during a miserable plague and full of sex and violence and somebody in admin will just delete the file, because their policy is to erase any mention of bad news. No bad news allowed. But I get so *tired* of all the false, maudlin, sweetness and light b.s. they print in the newsletter for us, uplifting feel good fluff, look at things on the sunny side, always on the sunny side, like everything is all right when everything isn't all right. It's not all right. Nothing is all right.

(Lights out except for a light on Martin's face, and two lights indicating the headlights of a car.)

Martin	I dream about my brother. In it, he's struggling to complete a difficult project, I don't know what it is, he has to drive some distance, and it will be dark when he returns and I'm thinking when did he start this new business, when did he start driving these distances, and why at night?—he's a terrible driver, the worst, and hates driving. I wake up realize it's only a dream, but I can't shake the compulsion to call and check on him, it's early but it turns out not early enough, he's already left for the day.

(Lights out on Martin, light up Irene's face.)

Irene	When I think back to the war it was hard, hard times, people lost, everything burnt, everything bombed—

(The sound of distant bombs.)

—buildings shattered, crouching in cramped bomb shelters in the dark, food rarer than hen's teeth, you learned not to waste anything. I was responsible for a squad of young women, recruited to serve as anti-aircraft gunners in Berlin, all of us teenagers, what did we know, we didn't know anything, but when the end came and it was clear things were collapsing, there were still some bitter old men muttering duty and honour and fight to the end. I listened to that nonsense, shook my head and told the other girls forget about it, walk away, do what you can for yourselves. Early one morning, just before dawn, I gave the word and we quietly abandoned the anti-aircraft positions.

I attached myself to a retreating motorized battalion and marched alongside them, raced to make sure that I would be captured by the British rather than the Soviets.

(Sound of bombs, closer.)

You heard from troops returning from the east, terrible stories of what happened if you were captured, nothing but rape and murder. Youngsters ten and twelve raped, grandmothers too old to walk, raped. Everything rubble and shattered concrete and smoke and murder and the Soviets advancing so quickly killing everyone. We had to cross the Elbe, get to the other side, the western side held by British forces. If we could arrange to be captured there we might survive. We took artillery fire half way there…

(Sound of bombs, close.)

…bombs raining down, smoke in the air, gravel spitting up, I took shrapnel slicing my leg one afternoon, calf to ankle, a shard lodged deep, I cut it out, bandaged the wound and kept going, it bled, but there was nothing else to do, we had to keep moving. Finally we arrived at the river's edge. Everyone had to make their own way. If we were captured as a unit, we would be delivered as a package to the Russians. I removed my uniform, folded it up, slipped into the river.

(Sound of a river.)

It was cold and dark swimming to the other side. I remember the strength of that swift current pushing. I bundled my civilian clothes and held them above my head so they would stay dry as I swam. I touched the far bank with my foot, felt mud and roots and reeds, grabbed a slick bush branch and pulled myself up and out. I had only just dressed and had begun walking when —

Soldier   —Halt!—

Irene   I encountered soldiers,

Soldier   Where are you from?

Irene   —and was captured. By the British.

             (Dennis shakes the pill container.)

Dennis   I watch the rain fall and think about taking my pills.

Martin   I watch the rain fall and think about my brother and my mother—

Irene   Have you taken your medication?

             (Dennis shakes his pill container like a maraca as he absently chants, and sways to the rhythm. As he does this, Martin simultaneously, and coincidentally, rises and stretches his back, and Irene extends and massages her stiff, cold hands.)

Dennis   One more pill. One more pill. Always, always one more pill.

             (Dennis shakes out a couple of pills into his hand and swallows them, ending their fleeting, impromptu, choreographed sequence.)

Martin	—and about how often my mother has been telling my brother, telling us both,
Irene	Don't move me. I want to die in my apartment. Just let me die in my apartment.
Martin	Not kill her, mind you, she doesn't want anyone to actually kill her.
Irene	I want to die in my apartment.
Martin	Just let me die.
Irene	I want to die in my apartment.
Martin	It's not a directive so much as a prayer. Just let me die in my apartment, and it's simply supposed to happen, and if only things were that easy, if only when things got desperate Death could be summoned like a repair person or pizza delivery, if only when you grew weary of life you could simply invoke Death like a hero of a bad novel to draw things to a tidy conclusion, but Death is incompetent. Summon all you want—
Counsellor	(*speaking into the phone*) Seniors' Health Centre.
Martin	—he never arrives on schedule. Hello, It's Martin Berenger, I was in some months back with my mother—
Counsellor	Yes, I remember.
Martin	She's deteriorated since then, and I just wanted to see if there's some further support we can access.
Counsellor	Right. She'll need another assessment.

Martin	Really? She's already been assessed several times.
Counsellor	It's a different assessment.
Martin	Right.
Counsellor	An assessment for mental capacity.
Martin	I thought that was what the previous assessments were for.
Counsellor	That's the protocol.
Martin	She won't want another assessment.
Counsellor	Nobody wants another assessment.
Martin	She hated the last assessment—
Counsellor	—They *all* do —
Martin	—she may not submit to another.
Counsellor	They can be stubborn.
Martin	Homecare has refused to care for her.
Counsellor	That's very unfortunate.
Martin	What am I supposed to do if she won't go?
Counsellor	Try to persuade her.
Martin	You don't know my mother.
Counsellor	If you can't persuade her, you may have to lie to her.
Martin	Lie to her.
Counsellor	Whatever it takes.
Martin	Really?
Counsellor	Really. Whatever it takes.
Martin	Thanks, bye.
	(Hangs up)
	Lie to her. Perfect.

Irene	I can't get up.
Martin	Let me help.
	(Lifts)
	There. Are you all right?
Irene	I'm so tired. I was kept awake all night by the *noise*.
Martin	What noise?
Irene	The yelling, the drinking, the carrying on.
Martin	*(dubiously)* The neighbours are pretty old—
Irene	Bottles dropped by the door!
Martin	—they don't seem like the type to hold parties—
Irene	Not them, your brother!
Martin	What? Where?
Irene	*Here*, in the condominium. He had people over drinking until all hours.
Martin	*Dennis?* Dennis hasn't had a party in his entire life.
Irene	The door was shutting, whang, whang, whang, and drinking and dropping those bottles. Clank, clank, clank! I saw them pushing their way in.
Martin	You saw them?
Irene	Yes.
Martin	Who?
Irene	The party Dennis brought over.
Martin	The party? Who were they?
Irene	I don't know their names! Six or seven people, maybe a dozen.

Martin	Where were you when this happened?
Irene	In bed.
Martin	Well, you can't see the front entrance from your bed—
Irene	I saw them!
Martin	You needed help from me today to get out of bed—
Irene	Don't tell me I didn't see them, I *saw* them, them with their noisy bottles and big boots and drinking!
Martin	Mom—
Irene	All of them right here!
Martin	Maybe you thought you saw them, or maybe—
Irene	Oh no, I didn't see it! I *can't* have seen it. I'm demented. I'm demented!
Martin	I convince her to go for her assessment. By lying to her.

I tell her the doctor needs to have a look at her leg, which has become seriously infected. Which I suppose the doctor will also examine. So, maybe not exactly a lie.

Let me buckle you in.

(*The illumination of street lights glide over Martin and Irene's face, indicating that they are driving. The marimba plays lightly as Martin speaks.*)

We drive to the Hospital in uncomfortable silence. Travel is a considerable hardship for my mother now and she is suspicious of what my brother and I are trying to do regardless of how we frame it. I don't know what will happen when we arrive, she may simply curse the doctors out, she may refuse to leave the car.

Dementia is described as a kind of 'decline' as though it were a leisurely descent down a gently rolling hillside. Nothing could be further from the truth. Dementia isn't a decline, it's a plummet from a precipice and as you fall you strike the rocky cliff face and each concussion removes another portion of who you once were. *Strike*—there goes your short-term memory, *strike*, there goes your ability to read, and strike, strike, *strike*, there's goes your recognition of places, of faces, of family, of history.

The medical team ask her a few preliminary questions, but when they inquire how she's enjoyed Homecare she launches into a blistering attack on their ineptitude, their youth, their disrespect, their inexperience, then segues into a celebration of sponge bathing and concludes triumphantly with an observation that the rigours of her escape from the Russians have left her capable of facing all real-life eventualities. The doctor nods and suggests testing my Mother's memory. My Mother—surprisingly—acquiesces. I'm stunned at how poorly she performs in comparison with her examination of only months before. There's almost nothing she retains past a few moments.

When Mom teeters out the door to have her mobility examined in the clinic next door, the doctor turns to me and says —

Doctor   —Your mother's physical health is seriously compromised.

She has a number of complicating infections, the most consequential in her right leg, but also on her left hip, that without dedicated, persistent treatment will only grow worse. I don't believe she can be counted on to remember to take the medication—

Martin   She can't.

Doctor   —And I understand that Homecare has been discontinued.

Martin   Unfortunately.

Doctor   Her hygiene is highly problematic, a contributing factor. Our tests indicate that her mental capacity has diminished so significantly that she no longer has the ability to make sound judgements. At this point she's at a considerable risk of harming herself or others. Our recommendation is that it's time to transition.

Martin   I see.

And by 'transition' she means it's time for my mother to abandon her home and furnishings and the entire life she's lived. A room will be prepared for her in the transition unit of the hospital within a couple of weeks, where she'll stay until a full time placement in a supportive living facility can be found.

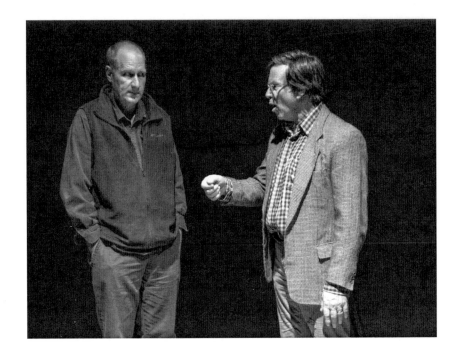

Two days later I receive a call saying that the Hospital has processed the doctor's recommendations, so we can make the transfer earlier.

(A light comes up on Dennis's face.)

Dennis   I had a dream last night.

Martin   So now, not a couple a weeks, but *this* weekend. A day away.

(The marimba presents a transition.)

Dennis   In the dream I was going to eat an apple, but it had a worm in it. When the worm crawled out of the apple, it turned into a green cockroach. So I crushed it with my thumb. I went to show Mom the squashed bug, but when I opened my hand it was a leafy plant instead that glittered and sparkled like emeralds. Mom looked at it and said, A bay berry plant! It can heal anything!

So I give it to her. And she's cured.

(Music ends.)

Martin   Are you going to drink your coffee?

Dennis   It's good, although I prefer Tim's.

Martin   I don't know if you've noticed, but things have kind of come to a head. When I brought Mom to the hospital for her last assessment they determined that she no longer has the capacity to live independently.

Dennis   I've spent almost forty years living with Mom.

Martin	On Friday I'll drive her to the hospital. She won't return.
	(*Beat.*)
Dennis	Okay.
Martin	You'll be on your own. Unless you'd want someone to live with you, or move in with us.
Dennis	Last winter Mom and I drove to Bowness Park together. I wanted to sit by the lagoon but it was too windy, so we bought a couple of hot chocolates and she and I sat in the car, the motor running, drinking our drinks, watching people skate, listening to Christmas music. When we returned to the apartment the wind had picked up and it had begun to snow.

I wouldn't be alive if it weren't for her. |
Martin	You understand she can't safely live in the apartment any more.
Dennis	I guess what you're telling me is I've failed.
Martin	What?
Dennis	I couldn't take care of her, that's what you're telling me.
Martin	No, that's not what I'm telling you. I'm telling you something completely different.
Dennis	You're telling me I've screwed up.
Martin	I'm telling you she can't stay in the apartment because it's too dangerous for her to stay, that it's beyond both of us. And I'm telling you it's dangerous for you. Every day the situation gets worse. It's affecting your mental health. The doctor's increased your anti-

depressants. You're depressed, and why not, the situation is totally depressing. She's awake nights, thinking who knows what, losing everything, forgetting everything, taking tumbles. You put your back out lifting her. She can't remember to take her medication. The toilet and sink are backing up, the entire place reeks, she won't let me help, she won't let anyone help, it's—

Everything's falling apart.

You can see that it's not good anymore, can't you?

(*Beat*)

Dennis	Yea.
Martin	Are you going to be okay?
Dennis	I guess.
Martin	We convene another early Sunday morning meeting. Mom detects something in the wind and sits ramrod straight in her chair as though confronting a jury, her eyes darting from one of us to the other.
	Listen. The head of the condominium board phoned to insist that we take action. She said that the condominium agreement states they have the right to evict you if the property isn't maintained. This just confirms what the doctor said at your last assessment—
Irene	Oh, I can imagine they are in touch with one another, they are in touch with one another certainly, the condominium board and Homecare and the government and they

	don't *give a damn* about us old people, they just want to kick us out on the street—
Martin	—Nobody wants to kick you out onto the street, Mom, and the government has nothing to do—
Irene	—Oh yes! That's what they want you to think!
Martin	—with the condominium board—
Irene	—But they are *busy* planning, and they have no interest in letting old people stay in their homes. They can make good money shoving them out and selling the property once they have stolen it—
Martin	—that's not what's happening—
Irene	—out from under me, once they have stolen it and lined their pockets—
Martin	—The doctors are concerned about getting proper care for you.
Irene	'Care for me!' I have more need of independence than of 'care'. At my age you learn to value your freedom, which everybody loves to seize from you. In all my years in the army I learnt to be useful with soapy water to clean myself, a bath or a shower can be wonderful but is not always attainable, but it doesn't mean you have to remain dirty. Now all they want to do is kick me out—
Martin	—No one wants to kick you out, everyone would rather you stayed, the condominium board would rather you stayed in your apartment, if you could maintain it, but

	you can't. This phone call is just another indication that you need help—
Irene	—Help? *Help?*— They don't know how to help. The help they send me is worse than useless. They send babies who don't know a blessed thing. They march into my home, track in mud and gravel, dump garbage in the sink.
Martin	Oh Mom. They don't dump garbage in the sink.
Irene	Come again! The plumber has been here how many times because they don't know how to treat a home, they send boys to shower me—
Martin	—They sent a man once. Once. By mistake—
Irene	—They steal from me—
Martin	—They don't steal from you—
Irene	—They do!
Martin	—and they apologized for sending the man—
Irene	—and then deny it. They push me, and punch me.
Martin	Who? When has anyone punched you?
Irene	They all do. They treat me worse than *a dog,* they hold my head *under the water* in the shower, and scrub and *scrub,* and I don't want any of it!
Martin	How would you know if Homecare works, you've never let them do anything. You won't let them clean the house—
Irene	—they can't clean!—

Martin	(*riding over her*) —you won't let them shower you, you won't let them make the bed, won't let them pick you up when you fall, won't even let them sweep up. If they're useless it's because you won't let them be of use—
Irene	—They don't send anyone qualified, they send *criminals* and *babies* who have never held a job in their life to *destroy* your home and steal from you—
Martin	—No one is stealing from you.
Dennis	—Mom, no one is stealing—
Irene	—They are *all, all* stealing from me!
Martin	—The dentures you thought were stolen turned up under your mattress. It's you that has dumped garbage in the sink, and in the toilet, and resulted in the plumber being called a thousand times! ! The money you thought you had lost you sent as cheques to charities.
Irene	—I never sent any cheques—
Martin	(*pulling out an envelope stuffed with dated cheques*) Cheques you signed and sent. Dozens of them. Throwing your money away, giving it to anyone. Before I took over your account you signed and sent these. And these! No one is persecuting you. The head of the condominium board has no connection to Homecare.
Irene	(*Talking over*) I would know if I had sent cheques, I kept the stubs and entered the amount at the back of the booklet, it's all, all in my purse—

Martin	—You hadn't made an entry in the cheque book for months! The situation at the apartment is unsanitary and dangerous and just isn't sustainable anymore. **Something has to be done!**
	(They finish talking over one another. Ringing silence follows.)
	It's time for you to move to an assisted living facility.
	Do you understand?
	Do you understand?
Irene	Kill me.
Martin	No one's going to kill you.
Irene	Just kill me.
	Kill me!
	(Beat.)
Dennis	I watched a TV show late at night, a man asked a woman do you want to control your feelings or do you want them to control you? I can't control what I feel and I'm not able to act on my feelings or I'd be sent to an asylum and they'd throw away the key.
	I own an old View Master, a plastic viewing machine with eye holes at one end to look into and a slot on top which you insert a flat cardboard wheel with tiny plastic slides, and as you depress a lever on the side, the disk spins about and the slides rotate around and around with each click of that lever. The oldest package of disks that I own is titled *Man on the Moon and the Apollo project*.

It's dated 1969. That's when I received it as a Christmas present. I remember presenting to my class in elementary school about the moon project and the lunar excursion module, about man stepping into the future, everything looked so clear, the astronaut climbed out of the excursion module into the darkness of the moon's rocky surface, click, he looked about at the stars and the Earth hanging in the sky and click, he planted a flag.

(He holds a View Master up.)

Here's my life in the View Master. Click, I'm born.

Martin   I don't know how to take her there.

Dennis   Click, I get diagnosed with schizophrenia.

Martin   It's two in the morning.

Dennis   Click, I wait in the psych ward in a hospital gown trying to figure out what to do with the rest of my crazy, useless life.

Martin   I'm awake in my bed.

Dennis   Click, I move back home with my mother and click, click, click thirty nine years fly by.

Martin   —and every time I think about the impending journey to the hospital—and it's impossible to stop thinking about it—I'm filled with dread.

Dennis   Click. She develops dementia and I try to help her but can't.

Martin   I try to organize my thoughts.

Dennis   Click. I transform into Judas and betray her. Click. I turn her out of the apartment. Click. Click. Click.

Martin

I have discussed with my mother how 'the transition' will proceed: that it will take time, that it will mean being registered through the emergency ward and signed into the transition unit until her assessment has been completed, and only after the assessment has been finalized will she be offered a placement at an assisted living facility, where they'll provide reliable medical care and a comfortable living arrangement.

And she's finally agreed.

But what does any of that mean, really? She's agreed, yes—reluctantly, unhappily—but will she even remember the conversation later this morning when I arrive at the apartment? Will she remember it *the second* we walk out the door? If she forgets or refuses to leave at the last minute, what am I to do? What if, at the hospital, she tells me she's changed her mind— if she turns about and shoves her walker out the hospital's main entrance? What should I do?

I lie awake turning these things over and over and over. At three in the morning I rise and take my place at the dining room table of my darkened home. I fire up the computer and prepare a list of the problems. There are dozens. I scroll down to a fresh page and begin a list of alternatives.

There are none.

Irene

When I first came to this country with nothing, I had never seen such vast stretches of land. On that long train ride west we passed field after field of grain where you saw no one.

No one. You saw forests, then more empty fields, then the train halted and one solitary person stood at the station, entered the train, a lonely battered piece of luggage clutched in his hands. Then the train rolled on again. After escaping a destroyed Europe, murder and smoke, and rubble and craters and ruined buildings, freedom. I realized I was free at last.

Martin   The day approaches and I'm sick with anxiety. Sick with dread.

I drive to the Y and run the track—

(He begins running on the spot.)

—past the treadmills, past the elliptical machines, past the seniors lounging against the metal railing chatting, past the stationary bikes, the balance balls, the chin-up beams, the seated leg curl and the stair master.

I try to think things through.

I try to find a way forward that presents a strategy that won't result in Dennis relapsing or my mother feeling betrayed.

I can't see a good outcome.
I focus on running.
I focus on breathing.
I wait for my brain to clear.

He continues running.

One more lap.

(The pill container shakes a quick concluding rattle. Lights down. The marimba plays.)

End Act One

CANTATA
RUMOURS OF MY CRAZY,
USELESS LIFE

Act Two

Darkness.

The sound of an intake of breath.

Exhale.

The sound of an intake of breath.

Exhale.

Martin   I arrive early, Dennis has already left for the
            day,

            The sound of an intake of breath.

            *Slowly a pool of light rises on Martin. The
            Marimba plays softly underneath.*

            I help Mom rise from her bed. She lingers,
            dressing as I lay out breakfast. We eat, drink
            coffee, clean up, then I say—

            It's time to go.

            Do you have your health card?

            *(She nods, indicates her purse which he is
            lifting from where it is hung on a stool.)*

Irene   Be careful with that.

            (She takes it from him.)

Martin   She loops the handle of the purse over her
            walker—

Irene	My whole life is in it.
Martin	—and straightens her shoulders.
	(*Music*)
	I open the apartment door, she sticks her key in the handle and locks it behind her. It's the last time she'll do that.
Irene	There!
Dennis	From the window I see the road stretching on. 'No trespassing' signs hang from a fence barring entrance to the road. Jack rabbits emerge like spies from grass clumps and ignore the no trespassing signs.
Martin	I buckle her in, enter, start the car. It's February, frost clings to branches, dusting the roadways, transforming the landscape to a pale, ghostly grey.
Dennis	They go where ever they want.
Martin	My mother relishes the ride.
Dennis	Hop, hop, hop.
Irene	Look at that.
Dennis	I pull my jacket tight as I walk to and then wait at the bus top. On one side the abandoned paved road stretches out to nowhere, constructed for who knows what reason, barricaded now with concrete slabs to prevent cars from entering. The road is painted with directional lines, though only rabbits and skateboarding teens use it.
	A bus lurches to a halt, I enter and it carries me deep downtown.
	I try to take my mind off what's happening.

	I avoid the panhandlers parked outside the Clubhouse, they always shout at me for smokes— I've told them a thousand times I don't smoke — and attend Circle of Friends. I help prepare lunch at Potential Place.
Martin	I park, walk to the entrance and borrow one of the hospital wheelchairs. I return to the car and help Mom into it.
Dennis	I know when I return home, Mom won't be there.
Irene	I can get into the chair. Myself.
Dennis	Not anymore.
Martin	We enter Emergency, where we take our place in line.
Dennis	Not ever again.
Martin	Mom is registered, has a green and white identification wristband snapped on. We park in the waiting room. Restless, my mother demands to know what we are doing here.
Irene	Where is this?
Martin	The hospital. This is part of the process of transitioning to a new facility that we talked about. Remember?
Irene	No.
Martin	The Doctor made recommendations that you come here, remember?
Irene	No.
Martin	This new doctor will meet you and formally admit you into—

(She turns away.)

But then she stops listening, turns away to watch a couple arguing, and I'm uncertain how much she has actually absorbed. I'm given, and fill out, a form describing my mother's 'lack of capacity'. It seems I've filled out a thousand of these. We are summoned by a nurse—

Nurse   Come this way.

Martin   —and conducted through the electronically operated entrance into the emergency unit, the doors clicking and locking behind us. I wheel Mom into a tiny cubicle like a tent, framed by floor-length shrouds of grey plastic curtain hung from a looping metal rod. Another nurse joins us, draws the curtains closed and holds out a folded hospital gown.

Nurse   Can you please put this on?

Irene   Why?

Nurse   It's for your examination.

Irene   Come again, I'm not going to put on *that*.

Nurse   I'm sorry, we need you to put it on.

Irene   No, I'm not going to.

Martin   A team of two nurses swiftly convenes to facilitate the procedure, and the curtain is pulled aside.

Nurse   *(To Martin)* Could you please step outside, thanks.

Irene   No. I said no!

Martin	She is, of course, filthy, having refused to shower for months.
Irene	No! Don't touch me.
Martin	The nurses don masks, smocks and gloves, and descend on her.
Irene	No!
Nurse	We're going to draw the curtain for a moment.
	(The curtain is closed once more.)
Irene	No. No.
	Get your hands off me!
Martin	After a brief, fierce struggle—
Irene	No!
Martin	—she is changed and clean.
	(The curtain is slid back.)
	She reclines on a cot, garbed in one of those especially inelegant open-backed hospital gowns, and waits.
	The fortunate thing about possessing a diminished memory, is that moments later she has entirely forgotten the incident.
	One nurse remains behind to gently comb my mother's fine hair, and pin it back—
Nurse	There.
Martin	—and in so-doing manages to restore some modicum of dignity to her.
	(They wait)
	Evening comes.
	Another nurse arrives to drop off a sandwich

wrapped in plastic, and coffee.

Time drags.

In the vestibule to our right a man vomits into a bucket, groans, and erupts again.

An alarm is mysteriously triggered—

(An alarm goes off)

and just as mysteriously quelled.

(And the alarm ends.)

The medical team argue in subdued tones about staff rotation, a nurse arrives to take my mother's blood pressure, and draw a vial of blood.

Irene	Ow.
Martin	The resident doctor joins us, asks mom a series of questions she doesn't really understand, records her answers that aren't really answers—

(She answers softly 'No' 'Yes' 'I don't remember' 'I don't recall' as Martin shares this section)

—signs the forms affirming her mental incapacity, and—

(She softly says—

Irene	There. *(indicating she has signed the papers)*
Martin	—formally admits her to the hospital. Another ten hours pass as we wait for a bed in the transition unit to become vacant, during which time Mom alternates grumbling, musing or catching a nap.
Irene	The days are certainly cold now.
Martin	Yes, they are.

Irene	What?
Martin	Yes, you're right, the days *are* cold.
	Very cold.
Irene	Long, and cold, and bitter.
	And the other day my foot became swollen, the same foot that took the war injury, and it *ached*. My God, it ached. But that's the thing about growing older—
Both	— it's not for the weak.
Irene	But, it doesn't hurt anymore.
Martin	Great.
Irene	At least I can hear sounds of humans here, alone at home conversations are not really possible, Dennis is so frequently out attending his groups and the medication makes him sleepy so early in the evening. You two used to be so loud when you were kids, racing about, jumping down the stairs, now he's so quiet.
	I enjoy the presence of another human being, though, and not always being solitary.
	Still I miss getting out, even driving to the grocery store, the Saturday trips to the farmer's market west of the city, not because I am a farmer, far from it, I grew up in Berlin, a city of millions of citizens.
	It's good to have family.
	(Pause)
Martin	Yes it is.
	(Pause)

Irene	Why am I here?
Martin	What?
Irene	It's nighttime. Why are we waiting so late?
Martin	We've talked about this. Remember?
Irene	No.
Martin	You saw and spoke with the doctor?
Irene	What doctor?
Martin	The doctor who asked you questions?
	And then you signed his forms? You'll be staying overnight to get assessed for a placement in the Transition Ward where you'll be tested to determine the level of care you'll require.
Irene	I don't want that.
	I don't want any more tests.
Martin	I know, but you remember what you said? And how they'll be providing care—
Irene	And I don't want any care from them.
Martin	But you remember when we discussed this, Mom?
Irene	No.
Martin	We discussed this—
Irene	No.
Marti	Mom—
Irene	— No, I want to leave.
Martin	Mom—
Irene	—I want to leave—
Martin	—Just listen—

Irene	Take me home, Martin.
Martin	That's not possible.
	And suddenly she understands in a way she hasn't before. I see it, I *see* the realization strike her like a bullet, the dawning that she will never return home, never have the life she had before, and it hits so suddenly and with such force that she recoils, and in order to maintain her composure and suppress her panic she focuses entirely upon her sandwich, carefully unwrapping and then folding the cellophane, stroking it smooth into a tidy, slick, compact square, consuming her meal, mouthful, by deliberate mouthful until, when the last crumb disappears and there is no more to eat, no more to unwrap, nothing left to defer her crisis, her body sags.
	(She sobs)
	Listen to me. Listen to me.
	Mom.
	It's going to be okay.
Irene	No, it won't. It won't.
Martin	It will.
Irene	No, no, no. Nothing is going to be okay—
Martin	—Mom—
Irene	—it's never going to be okay again. It's not.
	Who will take care of Dennis?
Martin	He will and I will.
Irene	Who will remind him to take his pills every night?

Martin	He will, and I'll help.
Irene	I've tried. I've tried to be a good mother.
Martin	We know, we know that, we're not saying you weren't. You were. This isn't about being good or bad, or succeeding or failing. It's about a really unfair, really terrible, disorder.

(*He holds her.*)

At six a.m. a bed opens on the seventh floor.

(*Martin releases Irene.*)

An orderly transfers Mom on a rolling metal gurney to a small, shared room in a ward for elderly patients. We slip past her new roommate who lies stiff as a fallen tree atop her bed, her head craned to one side, her mouth gaping.

The room is still except for the rhythmic gasping of her neighbour. My mother sits upright on her bed, her hands folded on her lap staring out the west-facing window. The sun rises after the long night, mountains glinting like teeth in the distance, a jagged line of rusty peaks cloaked in a dark bank of clouds. Wind abruptly gusts—

(*The marimba represents that gust and the snow.*)

—rattling the wind with tiny, icy pellets of snow.

Irene	It will be a cold morning.

(*The marimba offers a short transition.*)

Martin	I'm exhausted when I return home, collapse into bed and sleep twelve hours, but the

following day, early, Dennis and I rise to hold a cleaning party.

We throw open the windows of the living room to let in air. Grab old furniture that can't be cleaned properly—

Okay this can go, right?

Dennis	Yes.
Martin	And this?
Dennis	Yes.
Martin	We pitch old quilts, old bed sheets, old pillows, scrub counters and table tops, mop the kitchen floor, gather garbage bags full of debris, toss dirty clothes into the washer, we drag Mom's old mattress from her bed, up end it—

Lift!

Dennis	Okay.
Martin	—and toss it out. By the end of the session, the apartment still needs attention, but it's emptier, more orderly, more livable, and the odour is significantly improved.

Great.

There.

But when I leave Dennis, he has positioned himself on Mom's old chair, gazing out the same window at precisely the same landscape Mom did.

Hey. Don't you want to step outside for a bit? Get some air?

Dennis	No.

Martin	Are you just going to stay there?
Dennis	Yes.
	(*Martin lingers, wanting to say something.*)
	I have to take my meds.
	(*He delivers a quick shake of his pill bottle.*)
Martin	Her assessment comes back with a diagnosis of Mixed Dementia. A little bit Alzheimer's…
Doctor	Alzheimer's tends to follow a pattern of an extended, gradual decrease in mental capacity. The trajectory it follows is long and shallow.
Martin	…A little bit Vascular Dementia.
Doctor	Vascular dementia, on the other hand, tends to present like the steps of a staircase. Mental capacity exists at a certain plateau for a period of time, then there's a precipitous drop. There's no warning, nor is there any recovery from that drop. Skills that seemed assured one moment abruptly vanish. A new platform will appear stable for a period of time, until the next precipitous drop.
	Of course, that's just a profile.
Martin	So, how long?
Doctor	Each case is different. Maybe months. Maybe years.
Martin	The transition unit where Mom is kept until a supportive living unit is found corresponds almost exactly to purgatory. The average stay is supposed to be only weeks, but everywhere you see dispirited elderly patients, immobile, lingering in the hallways, collapsed in

wheelchairs vacantly waiting, watching who enters next, watching who leaves. In the background you hear the constant dispiriting soundscape of machines whirring, ventilators hissing, monitors and alarms beeping, calls crackling over the intercom and in some distant room, the disturbing faint echo of a crying patient.

We try to find a facility which will accept my mother.

Mostly, that process involves waiting for facility managers to call you back.

I drive to the apartment to pick up Dennis so that we can tour one of the facilities together.

Hello?

Dennis? Are you ready?

What's going on? Why didn't you answer the phone when I called? Why didn't you come to the door?

(Sees him.)

Why are you still in bed? Dennis?

Is something wrong?

Dennis	I don't know.
Martin	What do you mean?

Are you not…feeling well? It's one o'clock.

Have you eaten any food today?

Anything?

Did you take your meds?

Dennis?

Dennis	I don't know.
Martin	Let me look at your bubble pack.
	It hasn't been touched.
	Dennis, It looks like you haven't taken any of your pills. Not yesterday, nothing this morning. Did you take anything?
	(Pause)
	Did you take anything?
Dennis	No.
Martin	Did you check your blood levels?
Dennis	I don't know.
Martin	Have you been out of bed at all?
	(Pause)
	Have you?
Dennis	I don't know.
Martin	(*to himself, not angry, but rather, a realization*). Fuck.
	Come on, get up. Get up. You have to eat.
	First let's get some food in you. Here's an orange, can you peel it?
	(*He can't.*) Never mind, I'll peel it. Eat this. And I'll make some toast. There's some instant oatmeal. I'm going to make that.
	I thought you were going downtown to your art class? Did you?
	Dennis?
Dennis	No.
Martin	Did you call them?
Dennis	No.

Martin	Do you know their number?
Dennis	No.
Martin	Okay, we'll figure this out.
Dennis	Where am I?
Martin	What do you mean?
Dennis	Where am I?
	(slight beat)
Martin	You're at home.
Irene	The water is terrible, they try to get me to drink, but I tell them no, I won't do it.
Martin	It's just water.
Irene	That's what they *want* you to believe. They think I don't understand what they are doing, that I can't taste the poison they slip into it. But I can. And I can hear them, whispering in the hallway, preventing visitors from entering, no you can't come in. They want to poison me and they want me to die here alone.
Psychiatrist	I don't know what caused Dennis's latest episode of delirium, the CT scans of his brain are inconclusive, and its disappearance three days later is just as puzzling.
Martin	There's nothing that can be done to prevent a recurrence or predict…?
Psychiatrist	By the time you took him to emergency, he was already beginning to recover, so after the day spent waiting for a bed, observation in the ward didn't have much utility. What they observed was someone who was more or less capable.

Delirium can result from many things, physical trauma, diabetes, a high fever can produce a kind of psychosis. But nothing like that seems to have been in play with Dennis. And while his brain scan reveals some slight abnormality, there's nothing that should have produced that profound an effect.

Martin   So you don't know what caused it?

Psychiatrist Unfortunately, no.

Martin   Or when it will return?

Psychiatrist It's the mystery of my career.

(Lights down. A single flashlight illuminates Martin's face.)

Martin   In my dream I'm lying on my side in a bed.

(The marimba softly provides the score for the dream.)

The room is dark and cool. I'm comfortable but I don't recognize this space. It's small and rows of lockers line the walls. Three men enter without turning on any lights and start unpacking. At first I think I must be in a hostel of some kind, that other guests have arrived late. Then one of these men turns on a small flashlight, and the beam hits me, and I realize that the men are members of security. They are wearing some kind of uniform or overalls. They turn to me and two of them sit beside me—on benches of some sort maybe—and ask how I am. Only then do I realize, then, that over my blanket there are thick leather straps restraining me. I am fastened in. I tell them I am fine, but don't know where I am.

	Do you know why you are here, one of them asks. I reply that it must be because of something I did, dangerous or illegal, but I don't recall which.
Man	We know.
Martin	He doesn't sound threatening or angry, but there's something in the tone that is frightening
Man	Shall I show him?
Martin	The others agree and a screen drops from the ceiling. A video commences that I assume will demonstrate how I have offended.
	(Music halts.)
	I lie there in the bed, my bed, for some time after I wake, waiting for my crime to be revealed.
Martin	After three weeks I call Transition Services but instead of being put through to Moira, the woman I first spoke to, I'm transferred to someone new.
Claire	In the future if you have any questions about your mother's transition, you should speak to me, not Moira.
Martin	Okay. You're—
Claire	Claire.
Martin	I was trying to follow up with the person I spoke to last.
Claire	I will be handling your file, not Moira.
Martin	It's just that I spoke to Moira about the assessment, quite a while back—
Claire	The assessment has taken a few weeks longer than planned—

Martin	She was already assessed when she came in.
Claire	We wanted her reassessed and your mother's reassessment has been completed and her need for Designated Supportive Living (DSL) confirmed.
Martin	Great. So when can she move out?
Claire	You'll be sent a longlist of eligible facilities. Once you have selected a shortlist from that longlist, and delivered your shortlist to our offices, your mother's name will be entered into the data system. Following that, you can anticipate receiving calls of offer fairly quickly, some from the long list, which you may respond to or not, others from the short list which you have 48 hours to respond to.
Martin	How soon will we hear?
Claire	If you haven't heard anything within two weeks, contact me.
Dennis	When will she get placed and move out of transition?
Martin	Claire said shortly.
Dennis	What does that mean?
Martin	I don't know.
Dennis	One time we were all together at the condominium and a wasp flew in. I caught it with a Kleenex against the screen window. Ouch.

It managed to sting me, through the Kleenex. I still let it out. My brother said I should have squished it, but I don't hate insects they don't know any better, but I do hate people because |

	they do more than sting and they do know better. He said, that's where you're wrong. I said don't be so sure.
Martin	I return to the transition unit the next afternoon and find Mom asleep, seated in a deep puddle of urine. It's seeped through her pad and pants, pooled in her chair, and spread around her feet on the floor. Her slippers are soaked. She reeks. I inform the nurse at the desk, who glances up long enough to tell me
Nurse	I'll send someone.
Martin	Fifteen minutes later an aide arrives with a mop and bucket to mop the floor and a nurse arrives with a clean gown. She draws the curtain, helps my mother change and scolds her.
Nurse	Why didn't you press the help button?
Irene	I pressed the help button.
Nurse	I didn't hear it at the desk.
Irene	I pressed it.
Nurse	We'd hear it if you pressed it.
Martin	Even if she didn't press the button, someone has to check in on her.
Nurse	We do check.
Martin	Her slippers are soaked through.
Nurse	It's enormously busy at this time of day—
Martin	—I understand that it's busy—
Nurse	—And there are many patients on the unit—
Martin	—I know there are many patients—

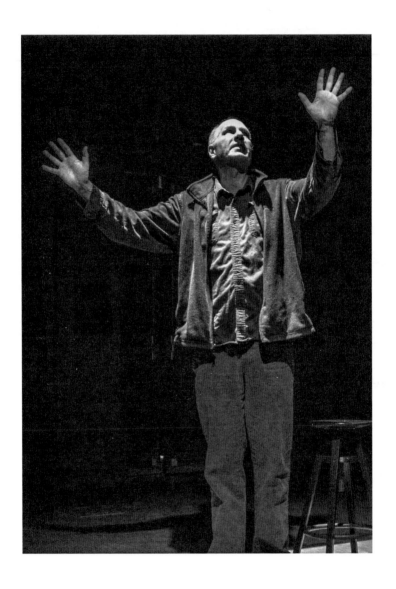

Nurse	—and every one of them needs our help.
Martin	Then help them.
	(slight beat)
Nurse	And she should have pressed the help button.
Martin	She has dementia.
Nurse	And you have to supply fresh disposable undergarments.
Martin	Pretty sure we brought a couple of cartons up earlier this week.
Nurse	Make sure when you bring them to let us—
Martin	—Isn't that them there?
Nurse	Where?
Martin	There.
	In the closet.
	Right there.
	(Beat.)
Nurse	Never mind.
Martin	Dennis—what happened to you?
Dennis	I was followed onto the c-train by a drunk.
Martin	The same drunk who went after you—
Dennis	*No*, a different one. You think there's only one drunk on the c-train? There are a billion drunk assholes who ride trains and live to make your life miserable.
Martin	When?
Dennis	On the way here.
	He kept saying he would fuck me up. He pushed me down. Some other passenger shouted at him, and I ducked out.

Martin	Did you press the emergency button?
Dennis	How? He was watching me.
Martin	Could you identify him?
Dennis	I'm not going to do that—
Martin	—The police could—
Dennis	—The police aren't going to do anything about that—
Martin	—Maybe he's known to them—
Dennis	—the police aren't going to do anything, they don't *care* about some random incident on the c-train between drunks and mental patients.
Martin	Were you wearing that hat?
Dennis	Yes.
Martin	Where did you find it?
Dennis	On the street.

(Martin removes it.)

Martin	Don't wear it anymore.
	Where's the hat I bought you?
Dennis	I lost it.
Martin	I'll get you a different one.
	Don't do that.
	Don't wear stuff you just pick up on the street. You don't have to do that. You don't know who wore it, you don't know if it's clean, you don't know anything about it—and it's red, and has this big, pompom, on top. It just makes you look.
	It makes you look.

Dennis	Like a target?
Martin	Yes. It makes you look like a target.
	(*He tosses it in the garbage.*)
	I'm throwing it out.
Martin	Three weeks pass without offers.
	(*Marimba plays*)
	I call Claire, leave a message, but get no response. Another week passes.
	Every time I visit the unit and see my mother shoehorned—
Irene	—they are poisoning me—
Martin	— behind the door of her room, hear her neighbour—
Irene	—poisoning me—
Martin	—in the adjoining cot weeping, see that my mother's dentures have been misplaced—
Irene	—every day, poisoning me—
Martin	—and no one has bothered to help her find them, see that a soggy blanket has been folded beneath her chair to prevent the urine from running around the floor, I feel I've betrayed her. Conversation with the staff proves fruitless, everyone's overworked, I know that and Dennis and I come up as often as possible, but the fact remains I convinced our mother to abandon her home by telling her that she would be moved to a better place, a safer place, a place where she'd be clean and cared for and instead she's been provided three meals a day in a hallway, and

left to marinate in her own urine. I realize that she can't remember the agreement she made, that she was reluctant to make it in the first place, and that if she could recall it now, she would almost certainly renege. None of that matters. The fact is, I said those words and she said those words and together they constitute an agreement, and I *have to find* a way to keep my end of the bargain. I phone and leave another message with Claire. Three days later, no reply. I begin phoning the facilities that are shortlisted and the ones in the quadrants that might be available, but am turned down.

Claire	(*Right away*) You're mistaken. No one is cherry picking.
Martin	I'm afraid they are, Claire, they take who they want—
Claire	Every SL 4 designated facility—
Martin	—*exactly* who they want, they take the easiest cases—
Claire	—blended private/public or solely public must accept clients with bowel incontinence.
Martin	I'm not arguing with you what is supposed to happen. I'm telling you what is happening. Which facilities actually do take clients like my mother.
Claire	They all are supposed to. Here is a list of available facilities.
Martin	I have that list already. My brother and I completed our selection based upon that list eight weeks ago. It was delivered to your office—

Claire	I haven't received it.
Martin	—but it is not useful to me if the facilities we've shortlisted won't accept my mother.
Claire	What makes you think they won't accept her?
Martin	Because we phoned them and they *told* us they won't, because of her bowel incontinence.
Claire	Every facility with the SL4 designation is supposed to handle incontinence.
Martin	That may be, but they said they won't. They have told me they won't. And not one facility has phoned with an offer in months and she was supposed to leave the transition unit within weeks and I can't leave her there any longer. So can you advise me which facilities will take her?
Claire	I cannot advise you because they are all supposed to take people with incontinence.
Martin	But they don't.
Claire	But they are supposed to.
Martin	But they don't.

(*A standoff*)

What are we supposed to do?

(*Music*)

I scrap the old list of facilities, start from scratch. Go looking again, lower my expectations, strike a new list. I make it my mission to find accommodation for her before the month ends.

(*Music*)

The Bow Valley Long Term Care Facility isn't pretty, isn't modern looking, is a bit run down, but it has its benefits. It's got vacancies, for one thing. It's located in a quiet neighbourhood, near public transportation —that's important, Dennis will be able to visit. It's a smaller facility, and maybe that means something. I find the large facilities cavernous and industrial. The staff-to-patient ratio is better than most. It also has a wide open central courtyard, with broad skylights that permit sunlight to warm all the inward facing rooms. Weeping figs, ferns, rubber plants and cacti fill the space, providing a bright, welcoming oasis. I stand in the middle of the courtyard and crane my neck to look up at the natural light streaming in.

Around me, clients quietly drink coffee as they assemble puzzles at activity stations.

Mom spent so much time in her apartment, gazing out her window at the trees. She'd like the courtyard.

Maybe this can work.

Irene   At last.

I complete the paperwork, and inform Mom she will be leaving the transition unit.

Irene   At long last.

Martin   An ambulance will drive you there in two days. You'll have to sign some paperwork at intake.

Irene   What do you want me to do?

Martin   Be nice.

(Soft music plays under the action.)

When I arrive the director escorts me to the physiotherapy room where a therapist measures Mom for a new walker while I fill out the necessary in-take forms and provide a voided cheque.

It's noon, and it's suggested that we go to the lunchroom as an introduction. Given my mother's unsteadiness, the physiotherapist advises that Mom use the wheelchair that she was brought in on, but it's a point of pride to her that she stand and use her walker and the physiotherapist acquiesces.

My mother follows a nurse to the lunch room, pushing her walker ahead, defiantly.

Irene   Hands off!

Martin   Fatigued by what for her is a long walk, she wobbles, and an attendant lurches in to direct, but my Mom is anxious, and her temper flares—

Irene   I said hands off!

Martin   It's all right, Mom.

Irene   It's *not* all right. Who does she think she is, putting her hands on me?

Martin   The attendant gives a quick shake of her head, indicating that it's not necessary for me to say anything, that this kind of response happens all the time.

Mom thrusts her walker into the dining hall.

(The sound of sixty heads rising)

—and abruptly the heads of sixty elderly

residents rise from their meals to study her.

(*She looks about considering the others. Music plays underneath.*)

And suddenly I'm overwhelmed by that feeling you get when you send your child to the first day of school and watch them cross the schoolyard. You know they're nervous, but you want them to be brave and demonstrate their best behaviour. You want them to be liked and accepted, to find friends and build a community. Only my mother doesn't smile at anyone, and she doesn't have a neighbourhood buddy to sit at her table, and this isn't school or a summer camp that she will grow out of or ever leave. This is the final stop.

(*Phone call*)

Martin	Hi Dennis.
Dennis	I visited Mom at the facility.
Martin	How was it?
Dennis	She begged me to take her home.
Irene	Can you get me out of here?
Dennis	I said I couldn't and she repeated it.
Irene	Dennis, take me home.
Dennis	She wouldn't stop.
Irene	Please.
Dennis	(*To her*) I can't.
Irene	Please.
Dennis	This is where you live now.
Irene	I *don't* live here. Dennis.

Dennis	I can't.
Irene	There's no place on the outside for me anymore? No place?
	(She begins crying.)
Dennis	Mom.
	(Transition music)
Psychiatrist	I've invited your brother to join us today. Are you okay with that?
Dennis	Sure.
Psychiatrist	How do you think things are going, now that you're living on your own?
Dennis	Not bad.
Psychiatrist	Not bad. What does that mean?
Dennis	I'm a little lonely, but…I'm okay.
Psychiatrist	And you? How do think it's working?
Martin	I'm not sure it's working. I'm trying to figure out how best to support Dennis. He's an adult. I'm his brother, not his boss. But it's his first time living on his own for nearly forty years. Mom prepared the meals at the apartment. She's no longer there. Before dementia hit, she kept the apartment in order. Again, no longer there. I came by the other day and the place is growing over top of him. There are garbage bags filled to the brim, crusty plates, crumbs, discarded paper and dirty laundry. I tidy up, but…
	Dennis has attempted suicide in the past. Every time he doesn't answer the phone, every time he disappears and doesn't leave a

message, I wonder, maybe I'll find him. This time, maybe he's dead.

He holds his cards close to his chest, he never wants to worry anyone. He says he's okay now, but he always says he's okay, even when he's not. I check in with him regularly, but maybe I won't catch it in time if things take a sudden bad turn. He's had these spells where he doesn't know where he is, or who he is.

What do I do with that?

What happens if he falls, or gets lost, or gets hurt?

Psychiatrist   What do you think? Is living on your own likely to be too demanding?

Dennis   I don't know.

I haven't tried to kill myself in a long time. Sometimes, I feel overwhelmed. I feel guilty about Mom. I visit her every day to make up for it.

I worry that I'm not doing things right. I worry that I'll be put into an institution next.

Martin   Why do you say that?

Dennis   I'm worried about it.

Martin   I'm not trying to put you anywhere. I *want* to support you. Mom's situation and yours are completely different. She was getting sicker and sicker and couldn't accept help, and fought with everybody. What could we do? It was only a matter of time before something terrible happened.

I'm not trying to control you or prevent you

	from living an independent life.
Dennis	I know.
Martin	I just worry that it'll be too much. I worry you're not eating well. You're diabetic, yesterday you had a single banana for breakfast, and what was it..?
Dennis	A wiener.
Martin	An uncooked wiener for dinner.
	I cleaned out the fridge the other day, everything I'd bought for him had gone rotten. There was a lake of decay and sludge pooled at the bottom. It took me an hour to clean it up.
Dennis	I know.
Martin	Flies flew out of the cereal box.
Dennis	I know.
Martin	I'm not trying to make you feel bad, but If mice got into the apartment, they'd be all over you.
Dennis	You're right.
Martin	And I'm not trying to run your life, but…
Psychiatrist	Would you accept help from Homecare keeping your apartment clean, ensuring that your medication is taken, keeping a bit of any eye on you?
Dennis	Yes.
Psychiatrist	How can you reassure Martin that you're not at risk?
Dennis	I don't know.
	Just, I'm not. Not now. I have something to

live for, something to prove. That I can make it on my own.

I can tell him if I have any dark thoughts. I've got a cell phone now, his number's in speed dial. I can call him.

Martin	Will you though?
Dennis	Yes.
Martin	You have to promise.
Dennis	I promise.
Martin	And you have to eat a real breakfast.
Dennis	Yes.
Martin	And something more than a wiener for dinner.
Psychiatrist	Maybe Homecare can help with that too.
Irene	Wait!
Martin	What?

I've taken my mother down to the garden, it's just an ordinary visit, when she abruptly announces—

Irene	I have to use the washroom.
Martin	And it seems to be urgent, so I lean down, place her feet back in the foot supports, push her in the direction of her room, along the way I catch one of the nurse's attention and ask her to give my mother a hand, they slip into the washroom together. She's gone what seems like a longer than normal time when the nurse returns out of breath.
Nurse	Can you help?
Martin	I follow her. When I step into the tiny washroom—

(*The marimba trills a rhythm of growing intensity*)

Irene	Get away from me!—
Martin	I am confronted by something—
Irene	Help!
Martin	—that looks more like a street fight—
Irene	Help!
Martin	—than a medical intervention—
Nurse	Hold her—
Martin	—My mother faces down three attendants, furiously batting away their hands—
Irene	*Let go* of me!
Martin	They're trying to strap a belt around her waist to lift her to the toilet from her wheelchair, but she can't figure out what it is they're trying to do—
	Have you explained to her…? Mom, they're trying to—
Irene	Take that *off* of me!
	Take that off of me!
Martin	Mom! Listen!
	She can't hear me.
Irene	Just help me up.
Nurse	Lean in!
Nurse	Take her under the arms!
Irene	I don't want that on me! Get that off me!
Martin	My mother darts a panicked glance at me.
Irene	Help! Martin, help! There are three of them and only one of me!

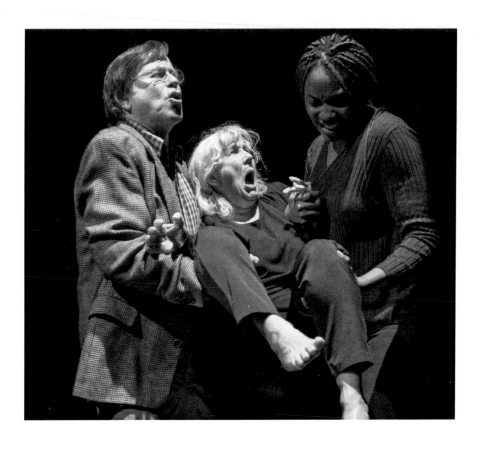

Martin	She shouts to me as though she's preparing to take them on in a street brawl, and needs to me to equalize the odds.
	I lean in to help lift her, but the whole operation is in flux now—
Irene	Ahh! Let go of me!
Martin	Five of us crammed into a tiny room only meant to accommodate one —
Irene	No! No! No! No! She's pinching me!
Martin	—and my mother keeps shrieking and slapping away hands like it's the fight of her life. Finally—
Nurse	Go on! Leave me with her!
Martin	—the senior nurse raises her voice above the din and orders all the other assistants to vacate the washroom. She and I stay behind. Mom briefly stops struggling, panting as she tries to recover.
Irene	*(Gasping)*
Nurse	Lift her by the waist strap.
Irene	*(Gasping)*
Martin	It's difficult because though Mom isn't heavy, until she gets her feet firmly placed there's a risk that she'll fall over. The nurse and I grab the lifting belt and—
Nurse	Lift!
Martin	—heave.
Irene	Ah!
Martin	I hold Mom there, mid-air, as she once more screams,

Irene	Ah!
Martin	—frightened that she can neither really stand nor sit. I kick the wheel chair out of the way.
Irene	Ah!
Martin	The nurse guides her backwards, and together, we slowly lower her onto the toilet seat.
Irene	(*Sighs.*)
	(*Beat. The marimba halts.*)
Martin	I'm soaked with sweat.
	I stand, straighten my back, and as I step into the hallway I think "Surely, surely it can't be this way every time she has to use the washroom?"
	Then when I finally take her back to her room, the senior nurse approaches me.
Nurse	Can you talk to her?
Martin	What?
Irene	Look at her, following us. (*To the nurse*) Get away.
Nurse	She won't get showered. She won't let us shower her. You see what she's like.
Martin	What do you want me to do?
Nurse	Try convincing to her.
Martin	What makes you think she'll listen to me?
Nurse	Try.
Martin	Mom.
	(*She turns to him.*)
	I know that this situation isn't ideal.

Irene	'Ideal'
Martin	But the food has been all right.
Irene	Sometimes. When they don't overcook everything.
Martin	But you would have a better relationship if you would let them clean—
Irene	Agh!
Martin	—you. Remember, I spoke with you about showering, and if you wore a shower cap that would keep your head dry, you remember? And I brought up several shower caps, have you tried putting on the shower caps I brought over?
Irene	Oh, I did—
Martin	Good
Irene	—but they pulled it off.
Martin	When did they—
Irene	—They *snatched* it off and they scrubbed and scrubbed and scrubbed until the water was forced through my skull and into my brain.
Martin	If they took it off, I'll talk with them—
Irene	—Oh, they'll tell you 'they don't know what you're talking about' and 'we're just trying to help', they're always sooo nice, but then they hold my head under water—
Martin	—I'm sure they don't hold it under on purpose—
Irene	—Oh they *do*—
Martin	—Why would they—

Irene	(*She shifts to another level of intensity*) —they do WHATEVER they want, it is like being in *prison* and they are worse than prison guards, they push me and shove me, and —
Martin	—Mom, it's not like prison—
Irene	—It is *worse* than prison, *worse*, I have no freedom, I get no respect, I am nobody, I am pushed and yanked and ordered about by nurses who treat me like a criminal, and I wish I was DEAD, I wish I was DEAD, DEAD and you wouldn't care if I was, the only one that loves me is Dennis—
Martin	—That's not true—
Irene	—And *you've never* cared for him—
Martin	—That's not true!
Irene	—Oh yes! *You* forgot all about him—
Martin	—I *never* forgot about him—
Irene	—and if the Unitarian Church—
Martin	—the Unitarian Church??—
Irene	—hadn't helped him—
Martin	—What are you *talking* about? The Unitarian Church didn't do anything—
Irene	—He would've been shoved out—
Martin	—Shoved out of *where*?—
Irene	—*Shoved out* and you wouldn't care, discarded, beaten, treated worse than a dog—
Martin	—What are you talking about? Your involvement in the Unitarian Church was totally beside the point, that the Unitarian Church did anything regarding Dennis's

	schizophrenia is just another of your delusions—
Irene	—Oh yes! That's right, you think I'm *nuts*!
Martin	—I've *never* called you that—
Irene	—That I'm incompetent, that I can't be trusted, that I'm garbage, nothing but garbage, garbage—
Martin	Stop it!
Irene	—garbage, garbage, *garbage*—
Martin	*Stop it!*

Okay, look, I've got to go.

And I shouldn't feel angry—she's old, ill, not herself, not her real self, but I can't *find* that real self, I don't know where its gone. And though I can remember a time when my mother was capable, and smart and kind, and loved us, I can't, feel it.

And instead I feel angry, cheated, and entirely lost. And for a brief time I wonder how I have possibly arranged a situation where everyone is dissatisfied and no one is happy.

(Christmas music. Very soft.)

So we attend the Christmas Dinner.

It seems a little premature, scheduled as it is on November 28th, but I suppose the administration want to guarantee that staff are present, and haven't yet booked their holidays. So, Dennis and I drive to the facility together, mount the stairs to the second floor, move past the moaning woman—

Moaning Woman	(*Moans ominously*)
Martin	—who stations herself like a sentry by the elevator door, and the man with the wild hair who always stares suspiciously at us, and find Mom in her room. She has selected, or had selected on her behalf a simple, burgundy blouse for the occasion, that matches her rust coloured slacks.
Martin	You look nice.
Irene	It was a lot of trouble putting it on. Where are we going?
Dennis	Downstairs.
Irene	Downstairs?
Martin	Remember? For Christmas dinner.
Irene	Is it Christmas already?
Martin	Well. Almost.
	Come on.
	We wheel her onto the elevator—
Moaning Woman	(*Moans*)
Martin	—and then out into the courtyard, which is draped with cut-out cardboard snowflakes—
	(*The marimba does something indicating snowfall, then transitions back into some other Christmas tune.*)
	—and long multicoloured streamers. Blue and white Christmas lights dangle and twinkle from branches above us. Round dinner tables draped in white linen stand

among the trees of the courtyard. We find a
handwritten place card— *Irene Berenger and
Family*—

Irene	Where do I go?
Martin	Here.

—at a table beneath the broad leaves of an
capacious rubber plant, and take our seats.
An elderly lady in an electronically powered
wheelchair arrives with a soft hum of the
motor, and she parks herself at the table
alongside her husband and adult daughter.

(Music continues playing in background)

A volunteer plays music in the background,
an eclectic mash up of pop tunes and
Christmas carols representing every decade
of music but the present.

Irene	What's the name of that?
Martin	What?
Irene	That instrument he's playing.
Martin	A xylophone?
Dennis	No.
Martin	What is it then?
Irene	Lebkuchen!
Martin	That instrument?
Irene	No! —these cookies. On the table. Lebkuchen They are the cookies you kids used to roll out at Christmas.
Martin	Oh. That's right! I remember.
Dennis	Yes. You mixed them in that big metal tub you'd cover in a dish towel—

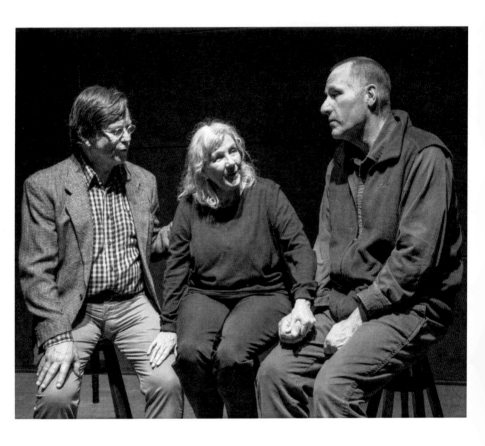

Martin	—and set outside in the snow overnight to chill.
Irene	Every winter.
Martin	Every winter. That's right.
Irene	You boys would roll and cut out cookies. Christmas trees and Angels.
Dennis	Sometimes we'd create our own designs. Cats. Fire hydrants. Death rays.
Martin	Right. That was a long time ago. (*Beat*) Well we better get settled. The meal is being served. Here, Mom, let me get your plate ready.
Irene	When the war initially broke out, I was just a child, sirens sounded and we rushed to a bomb shelter in the basement, huddled in the dark, listened to the explosions, felt them rattle the walls, boom, wondering when the next would fall and how close, boom, listening to people breath between bursts. Everyone was afraid. Afraid the end was coming. One old man, a veteran of the previous war, dug a harmonica out of his deep coat pocket. Music never sounded so good. (*Irena begins singing along with the music, softly at first.*)
Irene	The stars are brightly shining,
Martin	(*embarrassed*) Um.

	(*To Irene*)
	I don't know that it's a sing along.
Irene	(*She carries on, regardless*) It is the night of the dear Saviour's birth.
Martin	Mom?
Dennis	(*To Martin*) The others are doing it.
Martin	(*To Dennis*) But are they supposed to?
	(*Dennis joins in.*)
Dennis & Irene	Long lay the world in sin and error pining—
Martin	Who even knows the words—
Dennis & Irene	Till He appeared and the soul felt its worth.
	(*Martin reluctantly joins in.*)
All Three	A thrill of hope, the weary world rejoices, For yonder breaks a new and glorious morn.
	(*The song gradually takes shape as they sing together*)
	Fall on your knees! Oh, hear the angel voices! O night divine, the night when Christ was born; O night, O holy night, O night divine! O night, O holy night, O night divine!
	(*Music ends. Beat.*)
Martin	At the end of the meal, the dishes are cleared away and we're served hot chocolate.
Irene	That was a good dinner.
Dennis	It was fantastic.
Martin	It was.

	We wheel her into the elevator and up past the moaning woman—
Moaning Woman	(*Moans ominously*)
Dennis	(*To the moaning woman*) Merry Christmas.
Martin	—and back to her tiny bedroom.
	You look really nice.
Irene	So do you. Both of you.
	Thank you.
Martin	This is what I had hoped, that there might be a moment when, if we couldn't reverse things —and we couldn't, nobody could reverse things —we could at least slow the collapse. Hold on to each other for one moment.
	That's the last conversation I have with her.
	She lingers in bed one day, and is slightly off. Can't eat.
	She quickly deteriorates after that.
Dennis	She's stopped talking. When I visit she just stares into the distance and screams.
Martin	Vascular Dementia.
Irene	Eeeeeh!
Dennis	Mom, what is it?
Martin	Sudden, precipitous drops in cognition, and no recovery.
Irene	Eeeeeh!
Dennis	Is something wrong??
Martin	Within a few weeks, screaming is the only sound she can generate.

Then one afternoon I receive a phone call.

(In breath of eight, out with a puff. In breath of eight, out with a puff. In breath of eight, out with a puff. This continues throughout to the end.)

She's alone in her bedroom when I arrive,
stretched flat upon her bed, eyes closed,
one thin hand extended beyond the blanket
clutching the metal guardrail. Plastic tubes
snake up her nostrils. Her mouth gapes and her
breathing emerges in slow, painful gasps.

Mom?

I take her hand in mine. It's warm and dry and
papery smooth.

Her room is sparely furnished. There's no chair
beside the bed, so I perch on the hot air register
next to the bed and wait for the resident doctor
to complete his rounds.

Doctor	Pneumonia—
Martin	—the doctor tells me when he arrives. Apparently she took to her bed early last night, then wasn't able to rise for breakfast. He's seen—
Doctor	—this kind of thing happen many times,
Martin	—he tells me—
Doctor	—many, many times. It can progress rapidly—
Martin	—and it's hard to say how things will develop.
Doctor	It's possible that she will pull out of it.

But, she's ninety one.

Breathing. Inhale.

Exhale.

Martin	I call Dennis, inform him of the situation.
	Inhale.
	Exhale.
	My daughters sing to their grandmother, and she briefly opens her eyes and smiles.
	Inhale.
	Exhale.
	Inhale.
	Exhale.
Martin	At 2:45 am
	Inhale.
	She stops.
	Pause. Silence. No exhale.
	We hold a service for her at, of course, her beloved Unitarian Church.
	The service is fine, the singing incredibly poor.
	She was practical, and had already pre-purchased her cremation.
	On a cold, snowy January day we deposit her ashes in a deep, dark hole carved out of the frozen soil.
	And it's amazing to me that something can be both completely expected and at the same time such a jolt.
	I wish so many things. I wish we could have negotiated her transition to nursing care more easily. I wish she could have let go of her fierce desire for independence and accepted help. More than anything else I wish she could have been happier.

Dennis: Someday I will meet my Maker. And on that day, when that moment comes, I am going to punch him. He will never see it coming.

But then, God is supposed to see even the little sparrow fall, so he might be ready for me. He might smite me with a lightning bolt. But it would be worth it to take a swing at God.

(Dennis and Martin hug.)

Martin   The following day I sit with Dennis in the apartment. Him surrounded by her stuff, her furniture, her knicknacks.

Dennis   It's really just me here now.

Martin   Doesn't have to be that way. You could find a roommate.

Dennis   From my observation at Friends of Schizophrenia, that's got its own problems. Ted Buckley and Bill Weiser live together and are at each other's throats all the time. I couldn't stand the stress.

People think I can't do it. Live alone.

There was a time when I didn't think I could do it. Now I want to try.

Martin   I'm only minutes away.

Dennis   I know. I'm sixty-one. If not now, when?

Just for once I want to make them think I think.

Martin   Are you sure you want to stay here?

Dennis   Yes.

Martin   But, are you sure?

Dennis	I go to Circle of Friends, meet with folks at Opportunity works, Potential Place, Artists for the Poor. I attend coffee group. You and I get together.
	My days are full.
Martin	And you don't find the nights lonely?
Dennis	Mom's not here anymore. The trick is not thinking about things too much.
Martin	Or thinking about other things, maybe.
Dennis	Maybe. A marimba.
Martin	What?
Dennis	She asked.
Martin	Who?
Dennis	Mom. That's what that instrument was, that time at the Christmas dinner. A marimba.
	You strike something with a mallet.
	One hit is noise, a thousand hits, music.
	(The marimba plays, the mallets lightly striking the tone bars, as the stage fades to black.)

The End.

THE EXTINCTION THERAPIST

FOREWORD BY CHRISTINE BRUBAKER

FOREWORD
CHRISTINE BRUBAKER

NEW PLAYS ARE UPSTARTS. They can be unruly, petulant, hard to wrestle down and are always unpredictable. For me, a new play is an act of artistic heroism. Creating a world, a tangle of beings inextricably linked by a beginning, a middle, and an end—hopefully told within 120 minutes—crafting it all through squiggly black marks on a page is more work than the normal human will ever understand. And making it good? Well, that is another monumental task. It ain't easy. It's almost miraculous.

Fortunately, I am not a playwright, but I am a director, and getting a new play on stage is a mountain to climb. I had the good fortune to scale a most glorious mountain, directing, as I did, the world premiere of Clem Martini's play, *The Extinction Therapist*.

Clem Martini put his script across my desk back in 2018. When he described the story, I was intrigued: creatures on the brink of extinction grappling their way to their pending oblivion through group therapy. He told me it was a comedy and I paused, wondering what kind of world existed where a woolly mammoth, the Minister of the Environment, a Tyrannosaurus rex, and a smallpox virus could congregate. But that is the beauty of theatre, isn't it? We get to create these impossible worlds.

Personally, I've never liked the idea we must suspend our disbelief to enjoy a play—as if we somehow must put a part of our brain in 'park' to surrender to what's happening right in front of us. Rather, I like to think of theatre as expanding our belief. The best theatre for me invites me to see, hear, and experience the world differently. My heart and mind feel exercised, I feel bigger. As one of the most innovative directors in today's theatre, Anne Bogart, says, "a great play illuminates the dark corners of our psyches."

The Extinction Therapist does all this and more. It brings to light some very dark places. Yes, it is funny. Side-splittingly so at times, but one of its most powerful dimensions is a stark reckoning, a call for us as humans to face what we have done to our Earth. We are in a moment in time of rapid and exponential decline in our planet's biodiversity.

We are the cause and root of this impending disaster and Clem does not back down from this truth. The character of Smallpox calls Glen, the Minister of the Environment, "a weak spineless, writhing maggot', and names his crime by saying, "You could do something, you could, but you have chosen not to." As audience members, we are implicated in this. As a species, we'd better start acknowledging our interconnectedness to all of life, because ignoring it is at our own peril.

Clem has artfully given voice to this urgency through tender, fiery, and hilarious creatures. He describes them as "tinder" where the "slightest thing can ignite their buried emotions." And sparks do fly! Each creature has something to fight for—not just to remain alive, but to exist, to be seen, admired, recognized, and remembered. Just like all of us. So yes, while this is a zany story, it is also profoundly moving. It is a treatise on relationships, on love and all its insecurity, joy, loneliness, and longing. This play acknowledges us in our fear and trembling as we contemplate our own endings, even extinction, while also connecting us to that other feeling—an expansiveness, a hope, as we consider what's on the other side...the mystery of life.

Back to the making of new work. Inside this act of writing a play is the ultimate objective of seeing it produced on a stage. Here, there is a parallel, a similar fear and trembling, an insecurity and longing: Will the written word translate? Will the audience laugh and cry like we did?

Making new work is not for the faint of heart, hence the championing of the artistic hero who finishes the writing and the creative teams who forge it onto the stage. Over our few short weeks together in rehearsals for *The Extinction Therapist* as writer, cast, crew, and design team, we wrestled with the characters and story points, we fumbled our way down deep, dark design paths, only to realize we were walking in the wrong direction and had to turn back. We made trims and cuts, a full act, in fact, that is now our twilight-zone-ish epilogue. We fine-tuned the beats and moments during dress-rehearsals and previews. We worked, and worked, right up until just a few hours before our opening performance. We kept our sights on that light at the end of the tunnel, and when we arrived there, with a full house to experience the play out in the world for the first time, we collectively celebrated our journey. We all laughed. We all cried. We breathed a sigh of relief. And it was glorious.

—Christine Brubaker, 2023

INTRODUCTION
CLEM MARTINI

I wrote *The Extinction Therapist* because I spent most of the past decade feeling depressed and angry—and according to the UN's Intergovernmental Science-Policy Platform on Biodiversity and Ecosystems Services (IPBPS), I had every right to feel this way.

IPBPS indicates that one million species are threatened with extinction, that marine pollution has increased tenfold since 1980, and that a third or more of all amphibians are at risk of extinction. Furthermore, according to the UN's bulletin on The Environment Programme and the climate emergency:

> Climate Change is the defining issue of our time and we are at a defining moment. A wave of change is sweeping through the world with unstoppable momentum and… without profound changes to these sectors and a drastic cut to our carbon footprint, there is little hope to protect the planet from the worst effects of a warmer world.

Dire stuff. Obviously, I had to do something. Then, as I was sitting at my desk staring at my computer one afternoon, I heard a shrill voice off in the shadows complaining that 'The frustrating thing is that I can do nothing. What can I do? I'm a shrew.' Soon the other characters emerged from the darkness. As I crafted *The Extinction Therapist* over the subsequent years, I was supremely puzzled by the disconnect that existed between the high anxiety I felt, compared to the collective, world-wide response to climate change and mass extinction—surely an existential crisis—which could best be characterized as disinterested, distracted, inactive, and rife with misinformation and total, unadulterated BS.

Consider this classic quote from right-wing Breitbart News. "The two biggest human threats to wildlife in the last century have been a) Communists and b) Environmentalists."

Or this nugget of misinformation my own province's premier, Danielle Smith, shared when questioned about her party's views on climate change: "We have always said the science isn't settled and we need to continue to monitor the debate."

Or the observation that the former leader of the United States of America, Donald Trump, always a gold mine for inane and irresponsible remarks, offered: "The concept of global warming was created by and for the Chinese to make U.S. manufacturing non-competitive."

Clearly, we live in strange, strange times.

The cast of *The Extinction Therapist*, as they assembled, were a belligerent assortment of misfits and expendables, but between 2014 and 2023 these characters became my close confidants. I have rarely enjoyed living with individuals (and yes, when you work on play for nearly a decade, you actually do end up living with them) as much as I have enjoyed living with this particular support group. I loved the empathy and hope that Woolly Mammoth demonstrated, I relished the prickly volatility of Shrew, the sense of rage at injustice that burned in Smallpox, the vulnerability and total engagement with the healing process that T Rex expressed. And if Glen was no more competent than many of the politicians I've met, he at least had a sense of humour, a facet many politicians sadly lack.

This was the team with whom I shared my concerns when my city, Calgary, was choked with the obscuring woodsmoke of raging forest fires for weeks on end, when Fort McMurray burned for nearly a year, when Lytton, BC experienced a sudden spike of heat that made it the hottest place in Canada in recorded history, and then suddenly, tragically, incinerated. When the Splendid Poison Frog, and the Baiji Dolphin both winked out of existence in the same year, 2020, I mourned their loss with my *Extinction Therapist* cohort.

But why, you might ask, did I write *The Extinction Therapist* as a dark comedy? Because, let's be honest, the situation we live in is absurd, abundantly, astonishingly absurd. But also, because there is no energy to be found in despair. If we can laugh together, we can admit to one another that, yes, this situation is ludicrous—and terrible—and we must do something.

Time is running out, certainly, as Dennis tells Glen, but change is still possible.

—*Clem Martini, 2023*

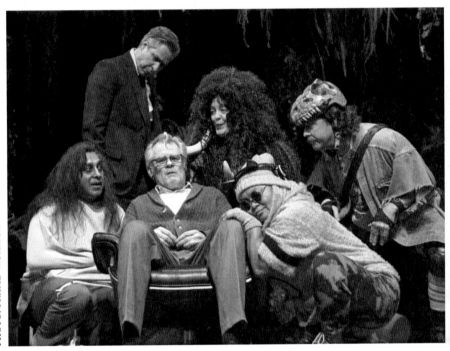

L to R: Anand Rajaram, Brandon McGibbon, Richard Clarkin,
Rebecca Northan, Karen Ancheta, Christopher Stanton.

CAST

PREMIERE PRODUCTION,
OPENED JANUARY 27, 2023
THEATRE AQUARIUS, HAMILTON, ONTARIO

CHRISTINE BRUBAKER — Director
JOSEPHINE HO — Stage Manager
REBECCA NORTHAN — Woolly Mammoth
and Joan Moreau
CHRISTOPHER STANTON —Tyrannosaurus Rex
ANAND RAJARAM — Smallpox Virus
KAREN ANCHETA —Nelson's Short-Eared Shrew
RICHARD CLARKIN — Dr. Dennis Marshall
BRANDON MCGIBBON — Glen Merrick
SCOTT PENNER — Set Design
LOGAN RAJU CRACKNELL — Lighting Design
JENNIFER GOODMAN — Costume Design

CAST OF SUMMER 2022
WORKSHOP, CALGARY, ALBERTA

CHRISTINE BRUBAKER — Director

JANE MACFARLANE — Woolly Mammoth
and Joan Moreau
HAL KERBES —Tyrannosaurus Rex
BRIAN JENSEN — Smallpox Virus
KIRA BRADLEY —Nelson's Short-Eared Shrew
DAVID LEREIGNY — Dr. Dennis Marshall
STAFFORD PERRY — Glen Merrick

THE EXTINCTION THERAPIST

CLEM MARTINI

Despite the therapeutic backdrop, The Extinction Therapist must move briskly. Members of this unique support group suppress deep passions, and though they strive mightily to conform to the careful protocols of therapy and encourage one another, they are tinder and the slightest thing can ignite their buried emotions.

Cast

Dr. Dennis Marshall—The Therapist. Male. A sixty-something rationalist.

Joan Moreau—The Therapist's partner. Female. Of a similar age to Dennis, but perhaps slightly more right-brained. (Should be double cast with either Woolly Mammoth or Nelson's Short-Eared Shrew).

A female Nelson's Short-Eared Shrew—tiny and intense. When she speaks, it is in short, quick eruptions.

A female Woolly Mammoth—warm and expansive. A lover, not a fighter.

The Smallpox Virus—male, pale faced, arms wrapped in a strait jacket, cold and imposing. Sees himself as an Alpha.

Tyrannosaurus Rex—male, possessing an immense head and tiny forearms. Experiences anxiety issues.

Glen Merrick—The charming-despite-himself Minister for the Environment, male, should perhaps remind one of a young John F. Kennedy. Early forties.

Note: The play is intended to be performed by six actors.

Settings

The action occurs in Dr. Marshall's comfortable office (leather chairs, oak desk and shelving, subdued lighting, framed degrees, interesting knickknacks), which is attached to his home. An unseen anteroom is employed, just beyond the office, on the way to the outer door. The anteroom contains a coffee machine and a small refrigerator, and it is there that snacks and refreshments are accessed by Dr. Marshall's clients.

An intermission must be taken after Act One.

THE EXTINCTION
THERAPIST

Act One

Scene 1   *Darkness. The sound of wind and rain. A spot of light warms and we discover Dennis. The clang of an alarm clock. A snippet of televised voice says, "...UN Climate Change Report Sounds Code Red..." followed by the eerie chorus of Rolling Stones Miss You...*

Shrew   The frustrating thing...

Lights rise on a Nelson's Short-Eared Shrew seated/crouched in a comfortable leather chair. Across a desk from her sits her therapist, Dr. Dennis Marshall in his chair, listening.

... is that I can do nothing. What can I do? I'm a shrew. Each day I'm famished. So *hungry* I can't describe it—(*apologetically*) it's my metabolism. Do you know that feeling? —that feeling where all you can think about is where your next meal is coming from? Where can I find my next meal!? All I want is a bite-sized frog or toad—and you never see them anymore. Amphibians. They're all gone. The number of times I've come across a frog in the last month I could count on one paw.

Dennis   You're focusing on the things you can't do.

Shrew   Yes.

Dennis   We've talked about that.

Shrew   Yes.

Dennis   What kinds of things can you change to make your life more pleasant?

Shrew	Nothing.
Dennis	Nothing? I don't believe that's what we've talked about in the past.
	(*Pause*)
	What have we talked about?
Shrew	I can't remember.
Dennis	(*Probing*) There's nothing you can do?
Shrew	No.
Dennis	Not even small things?
	(*Pause*)
	Could you alter your diet? Are there things other than frogs that you find pleasant to eat?
Shrew	Toads.
Dennis	Other than frogs and toads?
	(*Pause*)
	Are there things other than frogs and -
Shrew	*Yes.*
	(*Relenting*) Insects.
Dennis	Are there still insects available?
Shrew	Yes.
Dennis	Are there ones that you prefer over others?
Shrew	Yes.
Dennis	Could you choose to eat those more often?
Shrew	I suppose.
Dennis	What about your sleeping habits? Could you make your den more comfortable?
Shrew	I could shred more leaves.
Dennis	Yes?
Shrew	Use softer lichens.
	I've got to say those are pretty tiny changes.
Dennis	Lives are made up of pretty tiny things. Days are made up of minutes.

Shrew	Those changes will simply prolong my survival.
Dennis	Prolonging your survival is something.
Shrew	So. Enjoy my lingering demise. Savor the sweet melancholy of extinction. That's pretty crappy advice. Do you get paid for that advice?
Dennis	If you savour each moment, each day will be sweet.
Shrew	That doesn't change the fundamental problem.
Dennis	And what is the fundamental problem?
Shrew	I live within a limited range, and it gets smaller every day.
Dennis	That is not the fundamental problem.
Shrew	My habitat is drying, and food is scarce.
Shrew	That is not the fundamental problem.
Shrew	What *is* the fundamental problem?
Dennis	The fundamental problem is always the same.
Shrew	*Yes*, so what is it?
	(*Lights down on the Shrew.*)

Scene 2	*Lights up on the entrance to the office, as Dr. Dennis Marshal meets with another client, Smallpox. This client is a tall, severe looking figure, his arms bound in a white strait jacket. He enters and surveys the office skeptically.*
Dennis	Can I get you anything?
Smallpox	No, thank you.
	Is this where you meet all your clients?
Dennis	I operated out of a downtown office at one time. It was bigger, but I found I

could develop a more effective therapeutic environment here.

It's large enough to hold private sessions as well as run groups.

And of course, it's easier for me to get to the office when the office is my own home.

Please, sit down.

(*They both sit. Dr. Marshal raises his coffee mug.*)

And the coffee is better.

Smallpox	Why am I here?
Dennis	Everything transitioning to a final chapter finds its way here eventually. Everything narrows until, at last, it is seated in a therapist's office.

(*Smallpox considers this.*)

Smallpox	Regardless of time or distance?
Dennis	As far as I know.

(*Slight beat.*)

Smallpox	What do we talk about?
Dennis	Anything you like.
Smallpox	(*Grunts*) You handle many cases like mine?
Dennis	Every case has its individual nuance.
Smallpox	What do you do for your clients?
Dennis	We discuss feelings. Explore strategies for coping.
Smallpox	Really?
Dennis	Yes.

(*pause*)

Smallpox	And how does that work for them?
Dennis	I've received no complaints.
Smallpox	None?

Dennis	No.
	Were you expecting some?
Smallpox	What are your qualifications?
Dennis	(*Indicating the framed degrees*) You can see the degrees I've earned.
Smallpox	I don't mean professional qualifications.
	Have you ever had anyone close to you go extinct?

Scene 3	(*Dr. Marshall moves to meet his wife, who is in a hurry.*)
Joan	I thought you were going to be ready.
Dennis	I *am* ready.
Joan	You're not. Throw your coat on.
	You're going to be late.
Dennis	I'm going to be early.
Joan	How do you figure that?
Dennis	The clock says—
Joan	That clock in the hallway? It's broken.
Dennis	Broken?
Joan	Dennis, it's—
Dennis	Why—
Joan	—been broken for years.
Dennis	—didn't you tell me?
Joan	I thought you could read time.
Dennis	I read the time. Apparently, the wrong time.
Joan	You own a cell phone.
Dennis	Yes?
Joan	Can't you use it?
Dennis	I don't much care for cell phones, really.
Joan	What do you mean?
Dennis	You have to reach into your pocket, rummage

	about for it, drag it out, touch it to illuminate it—
Joan	My God, you make it sound like you've been asked to scale Everest. It's your *pocket*.
Dennis	And it's a waste of energy, the clock in the hallway operates on renewable kinetic power, generated by winding a key.
Joan	It doesn't work.
Dennis	Well, not *now*.
Joan	You should chuck it.
Dennis	It's an heirloom.
Joan	It's junk. It was junk when we got it.
Dennis	Junk that lasted decades, pretty good junk.
Joan	It doesn't keep time, pretty bad clock.
Dennis	Just drop me off at the train station.
Joan	What? I thought I was taking you and then you were attending the function with me after.
Dennis	Another appointment came up.
Joan	Why didn't you tell me?
Dennis	I forgot.
Joan	And you absolutely can't reschedule?
Dennis	You know I can't.
Joan	I wish to goodness you would keep better track of the things we agree we are going to do together. Now I'll just be that woman at the function, that woman at the function with no partner.
Dennis	We'll have another function, our own real function, not a made-up artificial function.
Joan	Fine, fine. Just, pinky swear or something, that you'll remember next time.
	(*They lock pinkies…*)

Dennis	Done. I'll remember.
	(…and release.)
Joan	Now *hurry* and throw your coat on.
	(Exit Joan, as…

Scene 4	*… Dennis turns to attend to another client.)*
Dennis	You mentioned…
	(Consults notes)
	… certain 'concerns' in your phone message.
Glen	Yes.
	I'm experiencing… unpleasant feelings.
Dennis	Can you describe those feelings?
Glen	Worry, anxiety, fretfulness.
Dennis	Do you have a notion about what makes you feel worried, and fretful?
Glen	My job, I suppose. Things to do with my job.
Dennis	What about your job?
Glen	There are others who are better at it than me for one thing.
Dennis	It's a big world. There are bound to be individuals somewhere who are better than you at your job.
Glen	You don't understand, I mean there are people who are better than I am at my job, *at work.* I'm the Minister of the Environment. And I'll tell you quite frankly, I am only barely on speaking terms with matters of this sort.
Dennis	I see. But that's easily correctable, isn't it?
Glen	I don't know that it is.
Dennis	You could, return to school.
Glen	I'm not sure I like the optics of that—Minister of Environment enrolls in undergraduate

	course. Can you imagine the kind of fun the press would have? "Minister receives failing grade in Environment 101."
Dennis	No one would have to know. You could do distance learning.
Glen	Between you and me, I was never much of a student.
	You don't have any drinks here, do you?
Dennis	Water or coffee?
Glen	I was thinking of an alcoholic beverage.
Dennis	No.
Glen	Right.
	(*pause*)
Dennis	What do you see as your principal role?
Glen	I'm not sure I understand…?
Dennis	What's the most important thing you do?
Glen	Well, I'm a politician, so I guess the correct answer would be serve the people.
Dennis	Right.
Glen	Except, that's not the way it is.
Dennis	No?
Glen	No, God no, my biggest most important duty is to lie to them.
Dennis	Really?
Glen	Look, the public don't want me to tell them, *your* economy, *your* lifestyle, *your* jobs, *all* your jobs, *all* the things you've been doing every day, *all* the things you've trained to do, *all* the things you love, are intimately, inescapably connected to screwing the world over. It's *you*. *You* are responsible. *You*. Not them. Not the one percent. Not somebody

else. You, you sorry fucker. The money you take home each pay cheque is based upon ensuring that the world today will be a little bit more poisonous tomorrow than it was yesterday.

Which is, more or less, the truth.

Dennis   Tell them that.

Glen   I'd be yanked from my cabinet position and lose my seat the very next election.

Dennis   Really?

Glen   And the candidate who replaced me would be someone delivering the same sorry BS I do now, which is that we will assemble an international partnership to fix these complex problems 'in the long term'. Again, total crap. Nobody is going to fix anything 'in the long term'.

Dennis   No?

Glen   No!—What *evidence* is there of anyone fixing international problems *in the long term*? We have a difficult enough time coordinating some phony baloney international endeavor like the Olympics in the short term which boiled down to its essential components is gathering a bunch of people together to play the equivalent of hopscotch every couple of years, and that totally tests our 'international cooperative' know how. So, if the truth won't get you elected, won't provide you with any influence to do anything genuinely good, even small things, even small good things for yourself, then what's the point in telling the truth?

Dennis	Do you believe that?
Glen	Yes.
Dennis	Honestly?
Glen	Absolutely.
Dennis	Then you don't need me.
Glen	What are you saying? What do you mean?
Dennis	If everything is okay, and you don't feel any anxiety or remorse, then-
Glen	But *that's* the problem! I know that I *shouldn't* feel anxiety or remorse. But I do.
	I wake nights sweating. Heart thumping like it's going to explode. Sweating, sweating, sweating—it's terrible!
Dennis	It's uncomfortable?
Glen	And dangerous. The public may not especially hate lying per se, but you must lie *fearlessly* because oh-my-good-god, they detest politicians who are insecure and they will take you to the ground if they detect weakness. The premier, my boss, can smell that particular flaw, it's uncanny, he's like a weakness bloodhound. I can sense him testing the air and selecting someone else more able than I am—Oh fuck me blind.
	(*He gasps*)
Dennis	What?
	(*He gasps once more.*)
	What's the matter?
Glen	Oh—
	(*Glen continues panting and clutches his chest.*)
	I'm finished. I can't breathe.
	(*He slides off his chair to the floor.*)

	I'm choking.
Dennis	Lean forward. Breathe into this.
	(*Dr. Marshal dumps his lunch out of a brown paper bag, and gives the empty bag to Glen.*)
Glen	My heart—
Dennis	Breathe into it.
	Just focus on inflating and deflating the bag.
Glen	I'm dying—
Dennis	You're not dying.
	(*He holds the bag to the Glen's mouth.*)
Glen	I'm dying professionally, the public will chew me up and discard me. I'm this close to being erased.
	And I *can't breathe!*
Dennis	You can. Out and In.
	Out and in.
	Long, slow, deep breaths.
	(*Glen is getting it.*)
	That's it.
	How often does that happen?
	(*Dennis helps Glen back into his chair.*)
Glen	Once or twice. A month.
	It's happening. More frequently.
	That's.
	Why I'm here.
Dennis	Keep breathing.
	Here's some water. When you feel you can, take a sip.
	(*Glen quickly drinks, then slips the bag back over his mouth.*)
	Breathe. Breathe. Good.
Glen	(*Putting bag down*) Oh god.

Scene 5	(*Joan enters, as Glen exits.*)
Joan	What are you doing?
Dennis	Fixing the clock you hate so much.
Joan	Don't worry about it.
Dennis	I'm not worried.
Joan	I mean don't tire yourself doing it.
Dennis	I'm not tired.
Joan	I can call someone—
Dennis	It's all right.
Joan	It's not. You've scattered parts everywhere.
Dennis	I'll clear it up.
Joan	You'll leave them there. They'll get oil on the carpet. There'll be cogs in the oatmeal.
Dennis	I'll eat eggs and toast.
Joan	Dennis, you're a terrible repair person, probably the worst handyman that ever was.
Dennis	That's a huge exaggeration. And if I were to call someone for every thing that needs fixing, it would cost thousands of dollars.
Joan	But they'd be fixed.
Dennis	They *will* be fixed.
Joan	Badly, incorrectly.
	(*He sits*)
	See? Now you've tired yourself out.
Dennis	I haven't tired myself out. I'm merely sitting. Everyone sits at one point or another. It's very common.
	The problem is you have no attachment to things.
Joan	They're *things*.
Dennis	Of course, they're *things*, if they weren't *things* they wouldn't be anything at all. That doesn't

	make them inconsequential things.
Joan	But my God, you have to place limits on things. Even Jesus who had seemingly limitless stores of patience, said you have to put a limit on the time spent on things.
Dennis	Where did Jesus say that?
Joan	Take my word for it, he said it.
Dennis	I don't think he did.
Joan	Luke 14:30, I'm paraphrasing. He said if you don't have enough money or time to finish building something…
Dennis	Yes?
Joan	Don't start. He said don't start what you can't finish, or people will mock you.
Dennis	Oh, Jesus was a bonehead, it's no wonder he took up religion instead of carpentry like his Dad. Can you imagine the kinds of things he built with that kind of attitude? People must have *dreaded* seeing him come by Jiminey, Joseph sent his boy Jesus over to fix the manger. Last time he came by it took him months to finish the door, the wind was blowing the place to bits, he kept repeating some nonsense about there being no point in starting.

Sell the clock,
Sell the bed,
Sell the house,
Sell the property.
We'd be hermits if you had your way,
less than hermits, hermits would look
comfortable beside us. We'd be mocked by
the hermits when they passed us by.

Joan	Now you're angry.
Dennis	I'm not angry.
	(*He drinks his coffee.*)
Joan	And you're drinking coffee again.
Dennis	It's not much coffee.
Joan	You shouldn't drink any. You won't sleep.
Dennis	I won't sleep anyway.
Joan	You could afford to throw that old clock away.
Dennis	I don't *want* to throw it away. A clock is a precious gift, a compass guiding us. A clock permits us to navigate these otherwise unknowable stretches of time.
Joan	Have you fixed it?
Dennis	Not yet.
Joan	Then we're still lost, aren't we?
	(*Joan exits as...*)

Scene 6	(*..Dennis starts moving chairs into his office. A Tyrannosaurus rex follows after him. The T Rex is very restless, and though he sits on occasion, he tends to pace.*)
T Rex	It's not so much that I can see the end. Everyone can see the end.
Dennis	You're early, our group session will be starting shortly.
T Rex	If there's a beginning, an end is implied—
Dennis	You may want to raise this matter when the others arrive—
T Rex	—I can understand that. Regardless of what's said about me, I'm not dim—
Dennis	Or, perhaps this is part of a longer conversation, that we might schedule later—

T Rex	—I get that. And I don't mean to sound ungrateful. I have many things going for me. It's just I don't feel…
Dennis	Yes?
T Rex	I don't feel, appreciated.
Dennis	Why do you think that is?
T Rex	Are you serious?
Dennis	Yes.
T Rex	Look at me. I'm the biggest carnivore in my biosphere.
Dennis	Yes?
T Rex	Nobody likes the biggest. I'm just the 'big, stupid, scary, largest carnivore.' And *I'm saying* it's not my fault. I didn't choose to be biggest. I didn't ask to be biggest. I don't *like* being biggest. Who would choose to be biggest?
Dennis	There must be some upside to being biggest.
T Rex	Hah!—there's *no* upside to being biggest.
Dennis	Not one thing?
T Rex	Nothing.
Dennis	You can see farther.
T Rex	Than who?
Dennis	The other shorter carnivores.
T Rex	How's that an advantage?
Dennis	You can see things—food—coming.
T Rex	Are you kidding me? It's not like we're all lined up on hillsides together and the first one that spots the prey wins. Those shorter carnivores are hidden in the brush closer where they can leap out quick. I have to run.

Dennis	And?
T Rex	I don't like running.
Dennis	Do you want to sit down?
T Rex	No!
Dennis	Do you want to talk about this when you're calmer?
T Rex	No! I want to talk about it now. I need! I need—
Dennis	What?
T Rex	I need—
Dennis	What do you need? Tell me.
T Rex	(*pacing more quickly*) What do I need? What do I *need*? I need so many things. I need understanding—
Dennis	You seem upset—
T Rex	I need to catch a break.
Dennis	Why don't you sit down?
T Rex	(*pacing*) I need slower running herbivore! I need nature to stop escalating the armaments race, I have bigger teeth, *they* develop bigger horns, I evolve bigger legs, *they* acquire thicker protective plates. And *these*! (*He shakes his short forearms in frustration.*) Are so *useless*!
Dennis	Here. (*Dennis pulls out the chair, and T Rex collapses in it.*)
T Rex	Really what's the point? I need a completely different system. And it's too late. It's too late.
Dennis	We have to focus on what we can change. You can live with it, live without it, or live beside it.

T Rex	And *that's* the problem—I'm living in it. All the way in it. I'm totally in it.
	(*A mammoth pokes her head into the office.*)
Mammoth	I heard shouting—
T Rex	I'm done.
Mammoth	It's five minutes past time for our group session. Can we come in?
	(*Sees the situation and half backs out.*)
	I didn't mean to interrupt.
Dennis	No, it's fine, we're just wrapping up.
Mammoth	Are you sure?
T Rex	(*To Dennis*) I'm good.
Dennis	(*To T Rex*) Stay after and we can discuss this further.
T Rex	Okay.
Smallpox	You're blocking the entry. Will someone shift him out of the way?
T Rex	You see? (*sadly*) Never any respect for the biggest.
Smallpox	The biggest *obstacle*.
T Rex	And *that's* exactly what I'm talking about.
Mammoth	(*to the others*) Come on in.
	(*A sudden flurry as the rest of the group enters.*)
Mammoth	Why are all these clock parts here?
Dennis	I'm fixing it.
Shrew	Fixing it. (*Eyeing the various parts skeptically*) Riiight.
Dennis	Let me move them.
	(*He sweeps the clock parts out of the way.*)
Mammoth	Is there another chair?

Shrew	Are we all here?
T Rex	I think we need another chair.
Dennis	Coming.
Mammoth	There was another client, wasn't there?
	(Dennis pushes a chair in from the next room.)
Dennis	There.
Mammoth	Do we need more?
Dennis	No, we're all here.
Mammoth	There was a woolly rhino at last group, wasn't there?
Dennis	Yes, she finished the program.
Smallpox	I find this one uncomfortable.
Dennis	Exchange it for another from the foyer.
Smallpox	Can someone bring in another?
T Rex	Another what?
Shrew	I'll get it.
Mammoth	You mean she 'finished the program'?
Dennis	Yes.
All	Oh.
	(Slight beat.)
Mammoth	I liked her.
Shrew	*(Dragging in a chair)* Where's the wooly rhino?
Mammoth	*(Confidentially)* Finished the program, apparently.
Shrew	Really?
Mammoth	Yea.
Shrew	Oh.
Smallpox	*(to T Rex)* Can we exchange seats? Last time I sat next to her it was like being caught in a woolly mammoth hair blizzard.
Mammoth	I was shedding.

	(*T Rex stands.*)
T Rex	Take it.
	(*They exchange seats.*)
Mammoth	It's seasonal.
Dennis	Okay. Has everyone found a place?
T Rex	Yes.
Smallpox	Yes.
The rest	Yes.
Dennis	Great.

(*They all join hands—Glen looks to Dennis*)
The words are on the sheet in front of you.
(*And, holding hands, they sing, to the tune of "We'll Understand It Better By and By[1]"*)

All   We are often tossed and driven
on the restless sea of time;
somber skies and howling tempests
oft succeed a bright sunshine;
in that land of perfect day,
when the mists are rolled away,
we will understand it better by and by.
(*They release hands.*)

Dennis   So. Good evening, everybody.
(*Others reply, 'good evening' 'hello'.*)

Shrew   Hello.
Mammoth   Nice to see you.
T Rex   Good to be here.
Dennis   Let's begin.
How are you?
(*Overlapping responses*)
Shrew   All right.

1 Tindley, Charles, 'We'll Understand It Better By and By', 1905.

Mammoth	Good.
T Rex	Fine.
Smallpox	As always.
Glen	Not bad.
Mammoth	And you?
Dennis	I'm well, thanks for asking.
	Please join me in greeting the newest member to our group, Glen.
Glen	Hello.
	(*All greet him.*)
Mammoth	Hello.
Shrew	Hi.
T Rex	Welcome. I think you'll find us only mildly intimidating.
Smallpox	Hello.
T Rex	Except for him. (*Nodding at Smallpox.*)
	(*Some mild laughter from others. Smallpox just stares.*)
Dennis	You're feeling at the end of your rope at work, is that right?
Glen	That's right. I don't know how I'm going to carry on.
Mammoth	You've come to the right place.
Dennis	Why don't we go right around? Provide a bit of an introduction.
Mammoth	Sure. Woolly Mammoth, the Pleistocene epoch. Struggling with climate change, environmental degradation, extended distance between breeding pairs. I'm finding it really, really challenging and am happy to be back among my peers.

Shrew	So happy to see you again!
Mammoth	You too!
	(*They fist pound.*)
Shrew	Nelson's short-eared shrew. Modern Era, but similar conditions to the ones she described, more or less.
T Rex	Tyrannosaurus Rex, late Cretaceous. Diminishing habitat, and increasing competition. I've found it nearly impossible to get three square meals since the onset of global winter.
Smallpox	Variola major, Smallpox. Modern era. Presently challenged to cope with my artificially, but severely limited, circumstances.
Glen	So, everyone here is…
Dennis	In a process of terminal transition.
Glen	(*A little intimidated by his peers.*) Quite a, diverse, group.
Dennis	Everyone adopts a physical form that will permit them to attend sessions.
Glen	(*Looking at Smallpox*) What, form is he?
Smallpox	What form are *you*?
Dennis	(*To Smallpox*) Hold on, he's new. (*To Glen*) We don't judge anyone on, or comment upon, the appearance adopted. Let's continue with a bit of a check in. What's on everyone's mind? What are you feeling? (*Slight pause.*)
Mammoth	I can begin. I find I really miss intimacy.
T Rex	Insecurity. Deep depression alternating with total despair. Lack of focus. The usual.

Glen	I feel anxiety.
Shrew	Struggling with loss. And I'm *hungry*—will there be snacks?
Dennis	At break.
Smallpox	The lack of genuine significance gnaws at me as a dog gnaws a bone.
Dennis	What do you mean by that? Significance?
Smallpox	Significance, real significance stems from agency over others.
	The riveting, electric thrill of knowing that someone's fate lies within your grasp. At one time I held that power, but that is no longer the case, and there's a delicious irony in my situation.
	At my zenith, at the very peak of my influence, I killed millions and enjoyed universal, unreserved deference. I exterminated everyone, levelled kingdoms and leapt continents, people fled my approach, yet *nothing* could outrun me—
Shrew	(*to herself*) Oh my god—
Smallpox	—my reach extended—
Shrew	—here we go—
Smallpox	(*turning suddenly on Shrew*) What?!
Shrew	The way he *gloats* and *goes on* about *the bodies*—
Smallpox	—What? I'm just sharing how I feel—
Shrew	—'oh the *millions* I killed'—
Smallpox	—which is a completely, one hundred percent accurate statement of fact—
Shrew	You know, you're not the only one that ever killed millions.

Smallpox	Oh right! (*A point that vexes him*) The bubonic plague!—that's who you're referencing, *everyone* talks about the famous *bubonic plague*, it's always 'Oh, the *bubonic plague*. It's so terrible. The bubonic plague. It's *so* deadly' but the only reason you even care about it is because you were a *carrier*.
Shrew	(*Slapping her forehead.*) Those were *rats*—rats were carriers. I'm a *shrew*! God!
Dennis	Let's try to remain civil—
Shrew	Sorry, I get impatient. (*To Glen*) It's my metabolism.
Dennis	And to be fair, the plague did, after all, destroy a lot of people.
Smallpox	Yes, yes, sure, but what was its kill ratio?
Dennis	I don't…know—
Smallpox	I *crushed* it everywhere I went. Diphtheria, same thing. Tuberculosis? Don't make me laugh. Cholera. Influenza. *Amateurs!* And now, look at me. I am a mere shadow of what I once was, and view with envy others I previously held in scorn.
T Rex	Envy? Tell me about it! I am filled with envy for everything that is going to *survive*— sometimes the most insignificant creature. Why them, I wonder, and not me?
Mammoth	(*mostly to herself*) I *know* that feeling.
Shrew	Sounds very familiar.
T Rex	And you want to know who I envy *most*? Snakes.
Shrew	Hey! If you're going to talk about snakes, I may have to leave.

	(*To Mammoth*) I lost my grandmother to a boa.
Mammoth	(*Commiserating*) Aw.
T Rex	Snakes. I'm serious. Every meal I eat, I work for. Searching, stalking, overpowering—the smallest snack is a foot race ending in a fight to the death. Then you realize that the future belongs to something that has never run a *single* day of its life! I'm telling you, snakes are the laziest sons of bitches you will ever see.

(*General laughter from the group.*)

No, really, have you ever seen a snake break a sweat? They spend ninety-five percent of their life, *sleeping;* the other five percent they spend *dangling.* How is that fair? For them, hunting essentially involves falling from a branch. I mean, c'mon, they don't even have to *chew.* While I'm busting my butt, they're sprawled on some tree limb, sleeping off their last meal. You watch, when I'm gone, it's snakes who will take over—and they'll have done it without even *waking up.* Tell me, *where's the justice?*

Smallpox	(*Darkly*) There is none.
Shrew	I regret that I didn't do more when I could have. I should have eaten more. Birthed more. Foraged more. Fought more.
Mammoth	(*Reminiscing*) Screwed more.
Shrew	Yes, sure, screwed more, definitely screwed more. Done more of *everything.* Moments lost forever! What was I thinking?

I'm young. Five months old, not even middle aged by shrew standards. I still have my figure. But where am I going to find a mate now?

Mammoth	That's exactly it.

Shrew	And it's not for lack of trying.
Mammoth	Tell me about it.
Shrew	I spend nights awake, yearning.
Mammoth	I've been there.
Shrew	*Yearning.*
Mammoth	*Yearning.*
Shrew	I've relocated my den three, four times, hoping I'd find the right somebody.
Mammoth	Left strategically placed spoor by the trailside, on the faint hope that the scent would attract male attention.
Both	*Nothing!*
Mammoth	And I daydream about sex *all the time.*
Shrew	Me too!
Mammoth	The little rituals leading up to it.
Shrew	The anticipation.
Mammoth	The *passion.*
Shrew	The *intensity.*
Mammoth	The *duration.* Those long, *languid,* unhurried periods of leisurely lovemaking.
Shrew	Meh.
	(*To T Rex*) What can I say—quick metabolism.
Mammoth	Now, I find myself obsessed with self-stimulation.
Glen	How do you define obsessed?
Mammoth	I, gratify myself, maybe five or six times.
Glen	A day?
Mammoth	A week.
Glen	That's nothing. If it was five or six times an hour, I'd be a little worried. Or proud. One of the two.

(The others look at him.)
You have to do something to pass the time during question period.
(The others look at him.)

Dennis   You masturbate during question period?

Glen   Well, not while I'm actually *answering* questions. Obviously. I'm *joking.*

Dennis   Perhaps this is a response to your anxiety. Would you like to address that sense of unease?

Glen   What can I say? My job makes me anxious.
I had no idea that the Environment portfolio would be such a *downer.* The Budget, yes. You expect the Economic portfolio to be depressing. The Health portfolio, oh Hell yes, you're dealing with arthritic grannies being shoveled into desperately crowded old folks' homes, Big Pharm, little kids with leukemia. But the *Environment*? I thought I would be the guy wearing the white hat.

Dennis   And you're not?

Glen   Nooo, heavens no. Every day is a complete insurrection. CEOs of major corporations in my face, hyperventilating, "what do you mean we can't stoke up that coke fired generator?" What do you *mean* we can't drill off *that* environmentally delicate shoreline, that we can't dredge *that* protected bog, that we can't level *that* grove of trees, *those* one hundred ancients; protected trees are, apparently, all that stands between them and total bankruptcy. And the *environmentalists* and *activists* and *shaman* and *Indigenous spokespeople* are just *beside themselves* about the latest threatened watershed or oil spill or aging atomic reactor, and they're strapping themselves to those gnarled trees, stripping themselves naked, chaining their scrawny, tattooed bodies to bulldozers, going on hunger strikes.

(He's hyperventilating.)

Dennis   Breathe.

(Glen takes a breath.)

Glen   God, everybody is so *bitter.*

Dennis   Why do you think that is?

Glen   It's like people can't reconcile the industrial, commercial and environmental concerns, but they're *all* part of the same thing. After all, big circle—the oil industry is just another part of the biosphere, right?

(With a single finger he draws a circle in the air. Beat. The others consider him.)

Shrew   I don't think you understand the term 'environment.'

Glen   I'm just saying we're *all* in it together. Let's everyone get along, am I right?

(He grins winningly at the group.)

Smallpox   *(Smallpox considers him as one might consider a bug.)* And there you have the terrible injustice of it all. At one point, I could have simply eliminated him.

Dennis   Remember the spirit of these meetings—

Smallpox   —And, really, when you consider it, I came *so close* to exterminating them. In seven hundred and thirty-five I swept through Japan and harvested nearly a third of the population. In the sixteen hundreds I scorched southern Europe emptying cities, sending survivors fleeing, broken to the countryside. I purged the Americas. Scoured China and excoriated India. Temples were created to worship me and sacrifices offered to appease me. Everywhere, people perished to burning fever, and bled from the eyes. In my most malignant form, skin turned jet black and slid off limbs in huge leathery sleeves. Bodies were stacked like cordwood in immense heaps ten and fifteen high. I stood astride the world, my power unrivalled, and killed by the hundred thousand.

Then—inoculations appeared and ruined everything.

Now, I cling to existence on the very verge— only two of my kind left. One, a sample in a closely guarded glass vial in Moscow. The other at the disease control clinic in Washington. My present survival hanging entirely upon the whims of others.

The resulting uncertainty is persistent, galling and humiliating.

That I should have possessed all that glorious autonomous power—and then, be relegated to the bluntest instrument of deterrence.

You.

Glen   Me?

Smallpox   All of you, your species, you fear me, yes, and yet are paradoxically drawn to me as well for the power I represent. And everyday I have to wonder—which of the two impulses is the greater?

(*Blows a hair from his upper lip.*)
Agh!—You're shedding again.

Mammoth	I can't help it. "Woolly" Mammoth—I'm built for the ice age and it's hot in here.
Smallpox	Ew. There are *hairs* on my collar!

(*He tries to blow them off.*)
Can you not *brush* your pelt before attending? Or shave?

Mammoth	You are *so* negative.
T Rex	It's true! I get that it must frustrate you being confined to two tiny glass vials, but could you at least *try* to be a little constructive in group?
Shrew	Are we going to take a break for a snack?
Dennis	Not quite yet.
Shrew	I'm starved!
Smallpox	Does someone have a lint brush? And hands free to help me?
Mammoth	And I am so *hungry* to be touched, it's maddening. I'm so tense!

It's no wonder I'm shedding, I'm coming into my cycle again. I need sexual relief and I haven't seen a male mammoth in, *months.*

I don't know that you can understand. We're built so differently. A trunk is an infinitely more sensitive instrument than a hand.

When two trunks coil about one another, every single receptor is completely engaged. It is a *sublime* sensation. Indescribably erotic. And as I grow older, I realize that the possibility that I will ever experience another close encounter of this kind grows more and more remote.

And to know that I will never again know

that exquisite, ecstatic intimacy. Do you have any idea what that's like?

Dennis   I can't imagine.

Mammoth   No! You can't. That's what I'm saying. You can believe that you understand what intimacy is, and yet have no idea.

I had a dream the other night, and it was, as usual, sexual.

There was some initial, imaginative, rugged foreplay. *Enormously* satisfying. My level of anticipation was so high. It was…It was—

(*She trumpets.*)

Glen   (*Too close and too loud.*) Whoa!

Shrew   (*Startled*) What the..?

(*T Rex Jumps up and roars his alarm.*)

Smallpox   (*Popping up.*) For the love of—

Dennis   (*Standing along with everyone*) Everybody!—relax.

(*Beat*)

T Rex   Sorry—just an autonomic response to sudden noise.

Mammoth   And I got a little carried away. My apologies. Won't happen again.

(*Everyone sits once more.*)

Dennis   Quite all right.

Mammoth   Anyway. To finish.

The dream.

It. Was. *Fantastic.*

I was enjoying myself thoroughly. It was sooo… soooo…

(*Dennis holds up a hand cautioning her.*)

Dennis   Remember—

Mammoth	No, I'm good.
	And then, suddenly—literally in an instant—he was gone. Vanished.
	At first, I thought it was just part of some sexual game, that he was teasing me, and I began searching. Everywhere. The whole time, totally aching with desire.
	And as I searched, I expected the ache to disappear, but it didn't. Instead, it intensified, until it became a genuinely physical, visual manifestation. I gained weight. My pelt became glossy. My belly inflated.
	It hardly seemed possible, but I concluded that I must somehow have been fertilized during foreplay. Contractions commenced. Intense. Protracted. I trembled and strained and groaned and all at once gave birth—to an immense shimmering cloud of the finest grey dust. A sudden wind rose from the north, and scattered it away.
Smallpox	(*Mostly to himself*) It's about death.
Mammoth	Pardon me?
Smallpox	It's about death. Am I the only one that sees it? All these dreams that you believe are about intimacy and sex are actually about death, it's always the same.
Mammoth	(*Hurt*) Oh!
Smallpox	What?
Mammoth	You don't have to be so *dismissive* of it— (*She cries.*)
Shrew	(*To Mammoth*) We understand, honey, it's okay.
Smallpox	(*defensively*) We're *supposed* to tell the truth.

Shrew	(*Then immediately to Smallpox*) Could you demonstrate a single *iota* of sensitivity? We're supposed to *support one another* you useless, oblivious germ!
Smallpox	(*Standing*) *Virus!*—a germ is a completely different thing, but what would a rodent understand about it?
Shrew	(*Standing*) Shrew, shrew, for fuck's sake, *shrew*! We're not rodents! We're not even in the same phylum!
Dennis	All right!
Smallpox	A bacteria can be a *germ*, a fungus can be a *germ*, a virus is a submicroscopic parasitic particle enveloped in a protein sleeve!
Shrew	At least I know the difference between a *rodent* and an *insectivore*!
Dennis	All right! That's enough! (*Shrew and Smallpox sit.*) There will be issues raised within our group which we return to from time to time.
Smallpox	(*More to himself than to the others.*) From 'time to time'?—give me strength.
Dennis	(*Dennis shoots him a look.*) That's not time wasted. Everything said within this circle has the potential to awaken something new in each of us—no matter how many times it's returned to. Are you alright?
Mammoth	Yes. I'm just feeling a little raw right now. (*Dennis turns in his chair and looks at Smallpox.*)
Smallpox	I apologize.

Dennis	And?
Shrew	Me too.
	(*Longish pause.*)
Smallpox	You know what my question is?
Dennis	No, what?
Smallpox	What about you?
Dennis	Pardon me?
Smallpox	What about *you*?
Dennis	I'm sorry, what about me?
Smallpox	What's *your* story? Don't you have anything better to do than listen to us soon-to-be has-beens bicker and share our woebegone yarns? It's late on Friday.
Dennis	I don't want to cut discussion off if it's productive.
	(*Beat*)
Mammoth	Right, I get that, but the point he makes is a good one, it's the weekend. The beginning of the weekend.
Glen	You have to admit, it is kind of strange scheduling.
Mammoth	There must be other activities you'd like to attend.
Dennis	No, nothing in particular.
T Rex	No?
Dennis	No, nothing.
Smallpox	Really? *Nothing*?
	That's pathetic.
Shrew	What's wrong with you? That's so unkind.
Mammoth	But it is, a little. Pathetic.
T Rex	I mean I'm happy enough to take a short

	break from the Cretaceous, but how come you're here this late?
Dennis	Because this is when our group session is scheduled and I am directing it.
Smallpox	But why? Why would you spend your Friday evenings in a room with a bunch of losers—
Shrew	(*overtop*) I reject that designation.
Smallpox	—Could there be a more precise, specific example of a loser-
Shrew	(*overtop*) I don't accept that designation!
Smallpox	—than someone who has lost *everything*, including every single member of their species—
Shrew	—(*overtop*) Speak for yourself, I don't accept that title.
Smallpox	—and who won't even exist in a short time, and so…whatever.
	(*Finally regaining the floor*) I mean, what is your problem?
Dennis	I don't see myself as having a problem.
T Rex	None? Even the greatest things on earth have *some* problems—are you saying you don't have *some* problems?
Dennis	I'm not saying I don't have problems, per se. I'm just saying we're not here, now, to discuss my problems.
Smallpox	Why are you so unable to talk about yourself?
Dennis	It's not really a therapist's job to talk about himself.
Smallpox	But surely you could share some kind of intimacy—

Mammoth	—some anecdote—
T Rex	—some reflection—
Smallpox	—even if it's just as a way of mentoring us.
Shrew	Yes, why are we able to let it all hang out, and you can't divulge a single thing?
Dennis	That's not what you come here for.
Smallpox	How many of you would like to find out what is troubling our fearless leader?
Mammoth	Me.
Shrew	Me.
T Rex	Me too.
Glen	Sure. If it's interesting.
Smallpox	And painful.
Shrew & Mammoth	It's unanimous!
Dennis	It would only be unanimous if I agreed, and I don't.
Smallpox	But—
Dennis	(*suddenly brusque*) So, let's move on. (*Brief pause*)
Shrew	Ouch. (*Brief pause*)
Dennis	Sorry, I didn't mean to be abrupt. Okay. The truth is that this time slot opened up as a result of a failure in my booking system. All right? I was supposed to attend an event with my wife. I was a little distracted and didn't enter it, so this time appeared to be open.
T Rex	It hadn't been entered in your computer?
Dennis	I hadn't placed the event in my day timer.
Others	Day timer?

	(*laughter*)
T Rex	Are you sure you didn't neglect to inscribe it on your *stone tablet*?
Smallpox	Who keeps a day timer anymore?
	(*beat*)
Shrew	What's wrong?
Dennis	My wife and I have separated. Have been for the last two years as a way of creating some space to sort things out. It's not unfriendly and I've always believed, completely believed, that we would reconcile and get back together. But I think she's met someone else.
Mammoth	You mean, she's had sex with someone else?
	(*Beat.*)
Dennis	Perhaps.
Shrew & Mammoth	*Ohhh.*
T Rex	Wow.
Mammoth	That's rough.
Shrew	How sad.
Glen	Very unfortunate.
Smallpox	Unforgivable, really.
Shrew	What would you know about it?
Smallpox	(*dignified*) I believe I, more than anyone else here, understand the implications of genetic betrayal.
Mammoth	What are you going to do?
Shrew	Yea, what?
Dennis	I don't know.
Smallpox	You have to strike back.
	(*General responses of dismissal and derision from the group.*)

Mammoth	Strike back?
Shrew	*Strike back?!*
Mammoth	What are you talking about?
	You've completely missed the point—
Smallpox	No, I'm afraid that *is* the point—
Mammoth	—*the point* in a relationship isn't to get even. It's to draw closer. To grow together. You have to woo her.
Shrew	Win her back.
Smallpox	Punish her.
T Rex	Maybe not punish her—
Mammoth	—for *sure*, not punish her—
Shrew	—what kind of fucked up advice is that?—
T Rex	—but I'd agree that you have to confront her.
Mammoth	It's not about confronting, it's about coaxing.
T Rex	It's not about coaxing, it's about candor.
	It's impossible to woo someone without first speaking truth.
Shrew	Never mind truth. You have to create trust.
Smallpox	Never mind trust, you have to set boundaries.
Mammoth	You have to make yourself available.
Shrew	Don't waste any time. Fast metabolism gives you an appreciation for moving swiftly. You live your life like a grass fire. My first partner lived a full, rich life and was gone in three months.
Mammoth	Really? *Three* months.
Shrew	I *know*—and I still miss him.
Mammoth	Love. Love is the only cure.
T Rex	For what?
Mammoth	Everything.

Smallpox	Total crap. If love could fix everything, we wouldn't be here.
T Rex	No, I think she may be right.
Smallpox	What do you know about it?
T Rex	What? You think the biggest can't fall in love? No creature is so large that they can't suffer a broken heart.
Shrew	I bet you miss her.
Dennis	Of course, I do.
Mammoth	Have you told her?
Dennis	We haven't been together enough over the last year for me to bring it up.
T Rex	Being the biggest, I think I can recognize that for what it actually is—a really *big* excuse.
Mammoth	Yea, that's just avoidance.
Dennis	No, I've respected her wishes for distance.
Smallpox	So—you've shunned her.
Dennis	Shunned her? I've hardly shunned her.
Glen	It sounds like you've shunned her.
Shrew	I agree.
Dennis	I haven't had time to raise a delicate matter that requires sufficient time—
Mammoth	Rationalization.
Shrew	Absolutely. Total rationalization.
Dennis	And she's been busy as well—
Mammoth	I know pain, and you're hurting.
Smallpox	I know anger, and you're angry.
Shrew	This is more than just anger.
Smallpox	Yes, but there's anger as well. Perhaps before anything else. You're *angry*, admit it.
Dennis	I'm experiencing many emotions—

Smallpox	Admit it!
Dennis	I'm angry, of course I'm angry.
Shrew	And sad.
Dennis	Yes! All those things.
Mammoth	Have you *told* her?
Dennis	No.
Mammoth	Tell her.
	Tell her.
	(*Blackout.*)

End Act One.

THE EXTINCTION THERAPIST

Act Two

Scene One	*Darkness.*
	A spot of light and we discover Dennis.
Joan	Hello?
	Hello?
	(*Lights rise on The Therapist's office.*
	Enter Joan.)
	Hello?
	I called...
Dennis	Sorry, didn't hear—
Joan	I didn't think you had a client, but wasn't sure.
	I thought I'd stop in and see how you're doing.
Dennis	I'm fine.
Joan	Are you?
	Your last appointment went okay?
Dennis	Yes.
	Listen, let me put things away, I can make us a bite to eat—
Joan	No, I only have a few minutes.
Dennis	Oh.
Joan	Yes, I just dashed in between things -
Dennis	You don't need to check on me.
Joan	I'm not *checking* on you -
Dennis	—I'm sure you're busy.
Joan	I can stop in for a bit. (*Beat*)
	Or can I?

Dennis	Of course, you can stop in, Joan, but I was hoping to have a longer visit to really talk. Things pile up when we don't talk.
Joan	Yes, well, I tried last time to have a longer—
Dennis	And I explained why I couldn't—
Joan	*You're* the one that's been busy.
Dennis	I called you back and left a message—
Joan	Three days later.
Dennis	—you didn't reply—
Joan	I came here. I'm here now.
Dennis	And how often does that happen?
Joan	It would happen more, but you have your sessions and your appointments to attend.
Dennis	The appointments are unavoidable.
Joan	I understand they're unavoidable. But you have to make time.
Dennis	Some of the appointments are non-negotiable—
Joan	—*You* have to make time.
Dennis	You can't just drop out because I have to attend—
Joan	It seemed clear to me you wanted space.
Dennis	I never said I wanted space.
Joan	You most definitely said you wanted space. You were the one that suggested—
Dennis	Come on, we *both* agreed that it would be better if we—
Joan	You couldn't even make it to the dinner we'd scheduled!
Dennis	An appointment came up. I told you—
Joan	—There's *always* an appointment or some reason—

Dennis	—and I didn't know it was so important to you.
Joan	You didn't *ask me* if it was important!
Dennis	And it wasn't a dinner—
Joan	Yes, Dennis, it was a dinner, food was served, I ate it, *alone*—
Dennis	—it was a 'function.' You said so yourself.
Joan	—I don't see the distinction—
Dennis	A dinner is a culinary event, sometimes romantic, sometimes social. A function is a necessary but essentially boring activity. You have biological functions, corporate functions, mathematical functions.
Joan	Well, Dennis, it was a function— (*Picking up her purse*) —a dinner function, that you chose not to attend. Because you were too busy. (*She exits.*)
Dennis	Joan!

Scene Two	(*Glen enters Dennis' office, takes a seat and continues his conversation.*)
Dennis	Do you have any close relatives?
Glen	No, no. Although my father's reputation lives on. Most years in cabinet. Most years Minister of Finance. He's quite famous, among certain other politicians.
Dennis	You mention your father often in our conversations. I haven't heard much about your mother.
Glen	My mother was sweet in a distant,

uninvolved, anaesthetized kind of way. My parents divorced when I was fifteen. I don't think I even noticed until I was seventeen.

Dennis   You followed closely in your father's career path.

Glen   Yes.

Dennis   That must have made him proud.

Glen   I suppose.

Dennis   I imagine he was supportive of you?

Glen   After his fashion.

Dennis   What do you mean by that?

Glen   People can imagine they are doing things for you, when in fact they are only serving themselves.

Dennis   Was that how your father operated?

Glen   Well. Let's just put it this way, my father ensured that every door was open to me, so long as it was a door he wanted opened.

Dennis   What do you mean by that?

Glen   One afternoon, toward the end of grade nine I walked into my father's office. I was attending a party later in the evening, and I had come to raid his well-stocked liquor cabinet. I knew he wouldn't be there. We had been informed that he was going 'to a conference.' That was a lie. He was flying to Florida to bang his office manager. I knew that.

I opened the door to his office and was surprised to find him on the couch, screwing another senator's wife. The senator was a close colleague.

She wasn't a serious liaison, of course. She

was just a diversion between the other more consequential affairs he embarked on. That was my father's addiction.

Anyway, he saw me, and saw that I saw them, and realized that he had an enormous problem. They both quickly threw on clothes. The woman exited.

We were left alone.

My father could see, in that moment, everything with absolute, awful clarity. He had been caught by his son, not only in an adulterous affair, but a highly compromising situation that could ruin him. He could see that he had made an enormous mistake. He realized he had to take decisive action.

He turned to me and said, "Don't tell anyone."

I was young. I was trying to stay cool. I said, "I'm just here for the booze."

He said, "I didn't mean for this to happen."

I didn't reply because I couldn't comprehend how you could find your way onto the couch in your office and into someone's pants, accidentally. Then he slipped me a hundred-dollar bill, and reached into his side cabinet where he kept his special stock, and handed me an unopened bottle of his Balvenie 40-year-old single malt scotch. I don't know if you're a scotch drinker at all, if you're not it won't mean anything, but that is a really beautiful scotch, the bottle was worth four or five thousand dollars, minimum. And he said, "Let's just you and I forget about this."

And I said, "I can do that," which was a lie.
And he said, "It will never happen again."
Also, a lie.

Dennis   So rather than apologize, he bought your silence. With a hundred dollars and a bottle of scotch, albeit an expensive one.

Glen   Yes.

Dennis   That must have hurt.

Glen   It was liberating.

Dennis   Liberating?

Glen   I had seen the truth. I no longer had anything to live up to.

Dennis   And so, you don't.

Glen   I suppose.

(*Beat*)

Dennis   And yet you remain in a career you were groomed for by your father. Doesn't that strike you as odd?

Glen   A little.

Dennis   Do you think, on one level, by performing duties you don't really believe in, care for, and can't be bothered to become competent in, you are indirectly punishing your father?

Glen   Punishing him?

Dennis   Yes.

Glen   No, that would be crazy. You can't punish the dead.

Dennis   True.

(*Pause. Dennis waits.*)

What's wrong?

Glen   I want to.
I want to punish him.

(*It's an uncomfortable thought. He puts it aside.*)
Something for me to consider.

Dennis   Yes.

Glen   Well. (*Consulting watch*) Times up—that's it for today.

I feel that was a, productive exchange. Don't you?

Dennis   Yes.

(*Glen rises to leave, goes to the door.*)

Glen   See you next appointment.

(*Glen tries to leave. The door won't open.*)

The door is locked.

Dennis   Yes.

(*Beat. He tries the door again. It still won't open.*)

Glen   Are you going to unlock it?

(*He tries the door again. Still locked.*)

I don't understand.

Are my payments late?

Dennis   Glen.

Glen   Yes?

Dennis   Is there something you want to tell me?

Glen   You mean beyond everything I've already told you?

No.

Dennis   You've slept with my wife.

Glen   What makes you think that?

Dennis   Haven't you?

Glen   No.

(*Beat.*)

Most certainly not.

Dennis	*Haven't* you?
Glen	No! How did you even come to that conclusion?
Dennis	Tell the truth.
Glen	It's a ludicrous notion. I don't know where you got it. Is there something I said? *Why* would I come to *your* office at *your* home and share my most intimate secrets with you for weeks, it would be *insane* for me to sleep with the wife of a man whose talents I engaged specifically to assist me. It would be too easy to discover. I would have to be an idiot.
	It's offensive, your accusation.
	And I'm offended. Very offended. No.
	(*Dennis continues looking*)
	No. Well, okay, yes, but I haven't slept with her in a long time. You're not going to shoot me or anything are you?
Dennis	Why did you choose my wife?
Glen	Well, she's attractive. And seemed to be, available. I thought she was single at first— you said yourself that you'd separated.
	I met her at the retirement party for some colleague or another and in a conversation I overheard her mention you worked as a therapist. And later, after, it occurred to me that I could use some therapy.
	And I liked her.
Dennis	And so?
Glen	I thought I might like you too.
Dennis	And you didn't see this as a problem?
Glen	I didn't intend for you to find out.

Dennis	You have to be *honest* with a therapist, Glen. That is the whole point! You have to allow yourself to be vulnerable. To be transparent. Did you not think that this might somehow come up?
Glen	I didn't think that far ahead.
Dennis	Well perhaps you should have.
Glen	I suppose. I'm sorry. I could really use a drink.
Dennis	*Stop* asking for drinks!
Glen	Right.
Dennis	That's part of your problem.
Glen	Right.
Dennis	You're not going to find an open bar in a *therapist's office*.
Glen	Right. Are you going to tell?
Dennis	No. I take an oath of confidentiality. And tell? Who would I tell?
Glen	I don't know. The press. My constituents. Her.
Dennis	I assume she knows that she's slept with you.
Glen	But that you know. About us. It was probably a mistake in judgment coming here.
Dennis	You think? (*Beat.*)
Glen	So, should I come back the same time next week?
Dennis	Are you joking?
Glen	No, this was good. I was confronted. *You* confronted me. Called me out on my misbehavior. I had to come clean.

I *never* have to come clean.

And I'm still standing.

So, I came clean, survived, and in my books that's a pretty good, pretty unusually good, outcome.

Come on—I screwed up, yes, but creating a safe space, allowing me to make mistakes and learn from them—That's your job, isn't it? Isn't it?

Everyone deserves another chance, right?

So, same time?

(*Beat.*)

Dennis   Yes.

(*This session ends as…*)

Scene 3   (*…we become aware that the group is in progress, a later date.*)

Dennis   Why be happy?

T Rex   Is that a real question?

Dennis   Yes.

T Rex   And you're asking me?

Dennis   Yes.

T Rex   If I knew that I wouldn't be here.

Dennis   Why be happy? Anyone?

Smallpox   Because feeling happiness flies in the face of reality and defies your actual grim, predetermined destiny.

Mammoth   Because happiness is a goal. Our essential life goal, I guess.

And because the other option is unhappiness?

(*Dennis tosses Mammoth a candy.*)

Smallpox	Did you just toss her a candy?
Dennis	Yes.
Smallpox	Is that what one gets for correct answers?
Dennis	Today, yes.
Smallpox	I don't know whether to be amused or insulted.
Dennis	Which one makes you happiest? How can we achieve happiness, in our most desperate circumstances? How do we achieve happiness on the brink of extinction? Anyone?
T Rex	I try to…place things in perspective.
Dennis	What do you mean?
T Rex	I have a bit of a tendency to fixate on being the biggest—
Smallpox	*Really?*
Mammoth	(*Cautioning him*) Now.
T Rex	Like, I've felt it was a more important tragedy that the biggest carnivore has fallen, but in these sessions, I've tried to challenge that perspective, and you know I've come to understand that it's *all* kind of beside the point. You were big? *It doesn't matter.* There's something coming bigger than you. You were important? *Forget about it.* You were fierce? Sexy? Smart? Deadly? *The world doesn't care.* It's found something smarter, sexier, deadlier. Get over it. *Get over it!*
Mammoth	I do a walking meditation to try to cultivate serenity. You asked how we achieve happiness in our most desperate circumstances—but times are always desperate, aren't they? The

	world is still beautiful in large and small ways. And I've already mentioned self-stimulation, I don't think that hurts.
Smallpox	I have comforted myself with the notion that if I am patient, eventually, I will be able to wreak terrible, agonizing retribution. But I'm coming to the sorry conclusion that time may have triumphed.
Glen	It's not *time* that has triumphed, so much as *technology* that has advanced.
Smallpox	Thank you so much for clarifying that point.
Glen	It's just important to understand that in this case it isn't so much fate you've encountered, as it is the advancement of knowledge.
Smallpox	Yes, I understand. Yes, yes, 'advanced technology', I get it.
	But I wouldn't get too cocky about that, I mean isn't that a bit of a sore point for you? Isn't it exactly *that* which keeps you awake nights?
Glen	I don't know what you're talking about.
Smallpox	Don't you? It's just interesting how your 'advanced technology' has circled back to bite you in the ass. Each new toy you invent has its own drawback, doesn't it? Yes, you can inoculate against diseases, like me, but there's always the next disease isn't there? Yes, your technology has provided you with ease and convenience but just consider the teetering mountains of disposable diapers, the towering pyramids of discarded cell phones, the immense, steaming continents of toxic landfills you've created.

Dennis	Give him time to respond—
Smallpox	Confess! Isn't there a teensy tiny part of you that wishes that I could be liberated for one minute, so that with one swift clean stroke, I might wipe the board clear and restore things to a simpler time?
	(*Shrew walks in and takes a seat.*)
Smallpox	But here we are talking shop.
Shrew	Sorry I'm late.
Dennis	Remember this is meant to be a conversation, so we want to allow time for others to reflect and address concerns.
Smallpox	Yes. Of course.
Dennis	We don't want to harangue.
Smallpox	No.
Dennis	The subject is happiness, and how we can achieve it. Glen? We haven't heard from you?
Glen	I don't know.
Dennis	Aren't there certain parts of your job you enjoy?
Glen	Not so much.
Dennis	Can anyone help him out?
Mammoth	There must be something. A small part of what you do that's fun or interesting.
Glen	Well.
Shrew	You can't be anxious the *entire* day.
Glen	Trips to foreign countries can be relatively entertaining.
T Rex	Are there colleagues you enjoy?
Glen	Oh please. Colleagues I enjoy? I mean, do those even exist?

(*Considers further*)

I appreciate training young people. We have a program for mentoring interns, and they're delightful, so fresh and hopeful. They dress so colourfully—The only spot of colour you'll see around the office most days. They're keen, limber, and much more optimistic, *so much* more optimistic than the previous generation. I mean, chalk one up for young people! And they're not inclined to gnaw on old grievances and waste their lives—and yours—complaining. They want action and hands-on experience, they want new sensations. I generally arrange to have an intern or two working closely with me and they're happy to receive instruction and I believe, with my years of practice, I have a lot to give. And I feel, you know, so much *younger* myself as a result of that close mentoring role.

(*An awkward pause.*)

Mammoth	I don't mean to pry. But these interns.
Glen	Yes?
Mammoth	Do you sleep with them?

(*Pause*)

Because it sounds in your description of activities a little like you might, and I don't think it's mentoring, exactly, if you sleep with them.

Glen	They learn skills as well—
Dennis	It's a breach of ethics if you have sex with your interns, Glen.
Glen	I've never received any complaints.

Dennis	Would you continue to employ them if they complained?
	(*Pause. Not wanting to concede the point.*)
Glen	Probably, not.
Dennis	Exactly. It sounds like, from everything you've told the group, today and in the past, that you're not really suited to your career. Are there skills that you have that you feel are portable?
Glen	Portable?
Dennis	That would transfer into another career.
Glen	I suppose. Soft skills.
Dennis	Soft skills?
Glen	I do pretty well in most social situations. People tend to find me charming.
Shrew	I find you repellent.
T Rex	To be fair, he's a human, you're a shrew.
Shrew	True.
Dennis	What aspect of your research catches your imagination most?
Glen	I can't say that I do too terribly much in that way. I make my decisions more on the basis of what I can infer.
Smallpox	*Infer*? But you don't know anything!
Glen	I don't have to know anything! That's the point. If I knew anything I would have to know everything. I'd have to *back things up*.
Shrew	You'd have to do research!
Glen	Yes!
Shrew	Which is your *job*.
Glen	Technically.
Shrew	Well do it!

Glen	Nobody wants me to do that.
Mammoth	What are you talking about? *Everybody* wants you to do that.
Glen	No, no, no! "Knowing" is a liability. It just prevents you from taking actions that are necessary but unpopular: firings, budget cuts, program closures, downsizing. But the problem is that I just can't keep track anymore. I've never been good at memorizing facts—and they're *facts*, things that hold some close connection to real things and events that you can Google or have your secretary look up—but *lies*, they're just in you, somewhere, and I can't remember them all anymore, and people get *sooo* angry if you lose track, just irrationally angry, like furious, like there was one elderly woman, very old, beyond ancient, a constituent, I told her, I don't recollect the exact wording, that I would try to have her property rezoned or some such thing so that some proposed, theoretical seismic exploration she was so worried about wouldn't occur, and then later, after the seismic testing had occurred and her ground water was found to be contaminated because it hadn't been rezoned—
Shrew	*Had you tried* to rezone it?
Glen	No, that's *the point* I made something up to satisfy her in the moment, try to keep up, but I couldn't remember exactly what I'd promised, and at a media scrum she confronted me, waded through the crowd, security just *caved* and allowed her to waltz through, and she was *so angry* I thought she

was going to kill me, she grabbed my lapel, with those bony, knobby, ancient hands, and kept shaking me, shaking me and shouting what's wrong with you, *what's wrong with you,* and now I simply tense up when I speak to the media, it's ruined me, without exaggeration, it's ruined me. I can't lie effectively, instead *I feel these hands, shaking me,* every time, and I worry that I'll forget what I said, so I try to keep notes, you know, right after an event—look at all these—
(*He reaches into his jacket pocket and a blizzard of post-it notes flutter to the floor*)
…but lying successfully depends on spontaneity, and you can't follow up *every single lie* with a reminder, and my anxiety levels just keep rising and rising—
(*He starts to hyperventilate. Dennis places a hand upon his head.*)

Dennis   Breathe.
(*Glen makes a conscious effort to breathe.*)
Keep breathing.
You have to stop lying.

Glen   Have you been *listening* to me?

Dennis   You *have* to stop. (*Dennis's fingers tighten around Glen's hair and he shakes him.*)

Glen   Ow.

Dennis   Sorry. (*Releases him*) Not just to others but to yourself. There is no other solution.

Glen   But—

Dennis   There is no other solution, Glen.

Glen   But—

Dennis	None.
Glen	But how will I continue to cope at work?
Dennis	You won't. You can't.
Glen	So, you're saying I'll have to resign.
Dennis	Yes.
Glen	Commit political suicide.
Dennis	Yes.
Glen	And do what?
Dennis	Something else.
Shrew	Anything else. I mean, I'm a shrew and even I can tell that you're terrible at your job.
Glen	It's all I know.
Dennis	Take a holiday. Develop other skills—
Glen	I don't think—
Dennis	I am going to tell you how your father died.
	(*Glen stops talking.*)
	He died in a drinking-related accident. Didn't he?
	(*Beat.*)
Glen	How do you know that?
	That's never been revealed to the public. Did you have someone research my family?
Dennis	I didn't have to. It's obvious. He had painted himself into a corner and every day he was reminded how tight a corner it was, and he drank to forget how hedged in he felt, and every day he painted another stroke.
	And, Glen, *you* are painting yourself into the same corner. Can't you see it?
Smallpox	I am going to sing a song

	Death, death, death, Death, Death, death, death, Death!
Mammoth	What's wrong with you? That's hardly appropriate—
Shrew	—and it's not a song.
Smallpox	It is.
Shrew	Where's the *tune*?
T Rex	There's no melody. Did any of you hear a melody?
Smallpox	A song doesn't require a *melody*, a rhythm is sufficient.
Mammoth	And the lyrics consisted of just one word.
Smallpox	It's a threnody, a very ancient form—you're all so conservative in your musical aesthetics.
Dennis	There is a war being waged in each of us, and a therapist is like a peace negotiator summoned to arrange a truce between the heart and the head. We try to awaken those two organs to the possibility of an agreeable ceasefire. Our heart wants us to be happy, our mind says the conditions are impossible and the clock is ticking. How do we negotiate a positive outcome?
Shrew	I am trying to be happy. I am trying my hardest to be happy.
Dennis	Does it work like that?
Shrew	What do you mean?
Dennis	Are we happiest when we try hard? Maybe we need to get out of the way and permit

	happiness to happen.
Shrew	(*frustrated*) Ohh.
Dennis	What?
Shrew	That's just lazy philosophy, it doesn't even constitute philosophy. It's a position. 'Just *allow* it to happen.'
Dennis	You don't agree?
Shrew	*Of course* you have to work for it. Even if it is simply clearing away the rest of the bullshit so that happiness can find you.
	(*Dennis tosses her a candy.*)
Smallpox	Did you just give *her* a candy?
T Rex	I'm trying to live with my conditions. Yes, I'll leave nothing behind. But nobody leaves anything behind. I'm okay with that.
Shrew	Now *you're* posing.
T Rex	What are you talking about?
Shrew	That pose.
T Rex	What pose?
Shrew	That one. That one right there. That 'Oh, everyone I know is dead, and I'll soon be dead too, but I'm not really concerned can you please pass the water?' That's total BS. You're scared senseless.
T Rex	Ha, you have no idea what it's like being the biggest. I'm not afraid.
Shrew	*Scared senseless.*
T Rex	I just have trouble sleeping at night— don't know why—
Mammoth	Because you're *afraid.*
T Rex	No.
Mammoth	It's okay. I'm afraid too.

T Rex	No! To tell you the truth, death will be a great release.
All	(*General noises of disbelief.*)
T Rex	I can't wait for it.
Smallpox	I'm with them now—that's a load of crap.
T Rex	Can't wait!
Mammoth	Not buying it.
Shrew	Me neither.
T Rex	You have no idea how freeing it will be! When I finally transition into the great beyond, food will be abundant—and all of it slow moving. I won't have to worry about horns or claws, or protruding spikes. I am telling you, life will be so much easier after I'm dead.
Shrew	Sounds like a delusion to me.
T Rex	It will be wonderful! Fantastic! I will be the happiest large reptile anyone has ever seen. No more fretting. No more *running, hiding,* or *fighting.* Happy, happy, happy! (*He contracts in his seat.*) Who am I fooling? There's not going to be anything. Nothing. Just an enormous void, an endless black gullet swallowing us whole, followed by an eternity of emptiness.
Smallpox	Relax. You won't feel a thing.
Mammoth	I don't believe that. I believe there is something after.
T Rex	What?
Mammoth	I don't know for sure.
Smallpox	Ha.
Mammoth	—And I don't need to know because I will guided into the mystery and I'll understand.

T Rex	Who will do the guiding?
Mammoth	The deity will instruct me.
Smallpox	Are you certain you will even be able to comprehend the deity?
Mammoth	Sure, because the deity will be a mammoth.
Smallpox	Nonsense. I have lived alongside the deity, and it is pitiless.
	The deity is dusk and ebony, river vapour and cold coal dust. The deity is the last silent breath a body sighs as it tumbles to the earth, the deity is death and decay and the dog devouring its master's corpse as it decomposes.
Shrew	The deity is tender and fierce and like nothing we've ever experienced.
	(*Standing*)
	Are there snacks?
T Rex	There were some salted nuts.
Shrew	Salted nuts. I don't know why we never have salted crickets.
	(*She exits.*)
Dennis	What about you, Glen, do you have any feelings about an afterlife?
Glen	I don't think I—
Shrew	(*off stage*) Oh!
	(*Returning holding an empty bowl.*)
Shrew	Empty.
	(*Looking darkly at the others.*)
	Someone ate *all* the nuts.
	(*She places the plate on the coffee table with a click and sits.*)
Glen	I don't think I've ever really had any serious—
	(*Suddenly Shrew pops up and kicks her chair.*)

Shrew	Would it hurt to leave *a few* behind?! Can't you think of the *others!!*
	(*She sits again. Beat.*)
Dennis	You seem out of sorts.
Shrew	Sorry.
	I mean, I appreciate these groups, but there is nothing that can compare to sharing your life with *someone* of your own kind.
	What happens when you no longer have anyone whose experience parallels yours?
Dennis	Do you feel lonely?
Mammoth	Sure. Yes.
Dennis	What about you?
T Rex	All the time. All the time.
Dennis	Isn't that a kind of commonality?
Shrew	Maybe I'm not making myself clear.
	We share *problems* here. And many of those challenges are shared challenges. I understand that. But nobody here, including you, can appreciate what it is like to be a shrew, in a shrew's body, with a shrew's fear and sadness and not a single other shrew in the entire world.
	That's my situation, and how can any of this help?
Dennis	Maybe we have to imagine a life beyond our identity, to a place where we all connect. You've (*nodding to T Rex*) mentioned that you're scared. How many of you are frightened?
Mammoth	I am.
Glen	Sure.

Dennis	How many of you long for the past and wish that you could turn back time?
Mammoth	Me.
Smallpox	Me.
Glen	Every day.
Dennis	How many of you contemplate death obsessively?
Glen	Me.
T Rex	I do.
Smallpox	I do.
Mammoth	Yes.
Dennis	But can we agree that everything that lives, dies? Right?
	That's inevitable, isn't it? So, what's the difference?
Mammoth	The difference is the intensity of the loneliness. Extinction isn't just your elimination, it's the annihilation of everything you knew, everything you cared for. You leave no traces behind, not even memories.
Shrew	It's the hopelessness.
	Yes, everyone faces death, but normally, there's hope that you will share your final days with others, hope that through your offspring you will leave memories behind, hope that your essence will carry on in subsequent generations.
T- Rex	The quality of the fear. I obsessively count the future in days. I have already seen others disappear before me, and I know on some level that eventually their fate will be mine.

	When will it happen? Tomorrow? The next day? I can't sleep wondering when exactly it will happen. Each time I close my nictitating membrane followed by my proper eyelid, I fear I'll never open either again.
Smallpox	Nevermind fear. What about fury? I'm supremely, enormously, pissed off.
Glen	(*interrupting to make his observation*) Now *that's* related to fate.
Smallpox	Can you *not* jump in so eagerly?
Glen	I'm just saying, your anger is a response to your fate, something that we all have to accept.
Smallpox	Please! (*Talking over one another*) Those are *my* feelings about *my* existence.
Glen	—Which are related to the events we have been discussing and extinction—
Smallpox	—*Yes*. My unfortunate and very undeserved extinction—
Glen	—Which is a response to fate!
Smallpox	Ohhh! *Yes*! everything dies, that happens, and yes that's destiny, that's *our* destiny, thanks for so glibly reminding me. But fate has nothing to do with the erasure of my kind. That, my sorry piece of squirmy, sticky protoplasm, is on *you*!
Glen	Me?
Smallpox	—you and your inept, incompetent, ill-considered meddling with *everything* around you and by all the deities real and imagined *where* is the accountability?

Glen	Hold on—
Dennis	Let's—
Smallpox	No, *you* hold on! You believe that you stand astride the foodchain, the glorious final product of a kind of benevolent evolution, but you stumbled up there, and what have you done since? You've destroyed *everything*! You don't know what you're doing, you don't know how to fix things, and all you can do is to continue your inept, ill conceived, *bashing about*!
Glen	That is simply projecting your bitter disappointment on a convenient target—
Shrew	I never thought I would agree with him, but he's right.
Glen	You too?
Smallpox	Finally, *finally*! Somebody sees!
Shrew	—He's totally right, you have screwed up big time—
Smallpox	Exactly!
Shrew	You've said as much! Here, in sessions!
	(*They continue overtop one another*)
Glen	—Oh, *here* we go—
Shrew	—and not just for you, for all of us—
Smallpox	—Yes, yes, *yes*!—
Glen	—Oh my god, you sound exactly like Green Peacers and the World Wild Life Federation demanding that I do something—
Shrew	—*for all of us!*—
Glen	—'...can you do something, please will you just do something...'
Shrew	—Well, why don't you *do* something?!

Glen	Because there's *nothing* to be done! Because it is impossible to reverse thousands upon thousands of years of human activity!
Smallpox	—You weak, spineless, writhing *maggot*, you mould, you sore spot, you *could* do something—
Glen	(*To Dennis*) He's haranguing.
Dennis	—Please sit down—
Smallpox	—you *could*, but you have *chosen* not to—
Shrew	—he's just telling it the way it is—
Glen	—More haranguing, so much haranguing—
Smallpox	—and if I could snap my bonds, if I could sever these restraints, if I could place my hands on you, I would scourge you for every second you excused yourself, every hypocritical justification, every absolution, every blind eye you turned—
Dennis	You must sit down!
Smallpox	—I would hold you to a *final account*, I would thrust a brilliantly bright mirror up close so that you could finally *see* how hideous you've become and then catching the searing light of the sun would focus that white hot beam and *incinerate* your sorry, insignificant form!
Dennis	—Everyone! *Settle!* (*silence*) This is supposed to be a supportive group.
Glen	And can I just say *that* was not very supportive.
Smallpox	It wasn't meant to be.
Glen	Well it wasn't.
Smallpox	And I have just told you that was not my

	intention!
Dennis	*Hey!*
	(*They stop bickering*)
	I have an exercise for you.
Smallpox	What kind of exercise?
Dennis	A trust exercise.
	(*Protests arise at once.*)
Shrew	Are you *kidding* me??
Smallpox	Really? A *trust* exercise? Oh no, no, no—
Shrew	With him? (*Glen*) Or him? (*Smallpox*)
Smallpox	I am *not* performing a trust exercise.
Mammoth	Come on.
Smallpox	No.
Dennis	It will only take a short moment—
Smallpox	Not with the likes of them!
Glen	Why not?
Smallpox	Because I don't *trust* you, that's why!
Glen	I make it a practice not to hold grudges, so you actually could trust me.
Mammoth	And me.
T Rex	Me too.
Shrew	Not me.
Smallpox	You see!
Shrew	I'd drop you like a rock. (*to Glen*) And you.
Dennis	It's not that kind of trust exercise.
Mammoth	What kind is it?
Smallpox	Whatever it is—
Dennis	It's an existential trust exercise.
	(*Beat.*)
T Rex	An *existential*—
Dennis	—trust exercise, that's right.

T Rex	How does *that* work?
Dennis	You'll see.
Smallpox	So, I don't have to fall into anybody's arms?
Dennis	No, no.
Smallpox	Leap off a table? Get lifted from the floor?
Dennis	None of those.
Shrew	Don't forget, *his* favorite hobby is killing *millions*—
Smallpox	Says the rat who acted as a vector.
Shrew	That's *it!*—
	(*She pops up.*)
Dennis	Sit down.
Shrew	—I'll show you rat!
Dennis	*Sit!*
	(*Dennis places a restraining hand on her shoulder and places her back in her chair.*)
Dennis	All of you sit back.
	Lean back in your chairs.
Smallpox	For what purpose?
Dennis	Just do it.
	Allow your heads to tilt towards the ceiling, take a moment, and relax.
	Everyone comfortable?
Mammoth	Yes.
T Rex	I'm good.
Smallpox	I still feel terribly uncertain about the particulars of this exercise—but I'm physically comfortable.
Dennis	Okay. Now, just breathe.
	Everyone can do that, right?
	(*A calm slowly descends on the group.*)

Breathe. Deeply. Slowly.

In.

And out.

Again.

In.

(*We become aware of the slow, rhythmic, collective intake of breath from the entire group in unison.*)

And out.

(*And the unified exhalation of breath.*)

And in.

(*Again, rhythmic. Deep. They carry on, in and out.*)

Now.

Everyone is calm? Relaxed?

All	Yes.
Dennis	Good. Keep breathing.

In.

And out.

Keep breathing.

Imagine your essence. The very core of who you are.

Powerful. Vital.

Imagine it has been distilled into something so tiny that it can slip out of your body on a single exhaled breath.

(*He reaches into a desk drawer and withdraws a small black box. He sets the box on his desktop and then takes the lid off the box. From within the box he pulls the tiniest sliver of gossamer, which he holds over the shrew. He releases it and it slowly drifts downward. Shrew*) *breathes out, and her breath lifts the filament high above her. A beam of light catches it, where it floats brilliantly in the air.)*

Dennis   There it is.

(The filament hangs, glowing, in the air.)

Free.

Unworried.

Unconfined.

(It starts to drop, but as Shrew exhales, it is buoyed upward once again. The soft but persistent, rhythmic breathing of the entire group continues in the background.)

It floats, bobbing, just slightly above your head. Where you can view and consider it for all its merits and flaws. A brilliant, eternal, point of light.

(It slowly begins to sink once again. With a puff it returns up high. It begins to drop.)

You have only one job now.

Keep it suspended.

(The shrew puffs and the gossamer floats back up.)

Imagine that is not only something that exists, but that it is something you have agency over.

Guide it to the individual immediately next to you. You have no fear, because you know that that we are here for each other, and it will be cared for and supported in a gentle, controlled orbit clockwise around the circle.

That's *why* you are here, why we are all here. To care for one another. And each supporting breath sustains and exposes some new facet of your essence.

As it goes around, you are able to view it with greater and greater clarity, and you begin to understand who you are, and what you need.

(*The shrew puffs the gossamer. It floats in a graceful arc and begins to descend in front of Mammoth.*)

Mammoth	It's dropping!—
Dennis	Not to worry, its descent is gradual, and the slightest breath can elevate it. And from this perspective, disconnected, you can step outside yourself, assess it and consider what it truly requires.

(*Mammoth exhales and the gossamer filament lifts.*)

(*Glen blows lightly.*)

Rising. Rising. Falling. Buoyant. Free of care. And as it continues its cycle, consider how exquisite it is.

(*T Rex puffs.*)

Rising. Falling. Powerful and resilient.

(*Smallpox puffs.*)

Coming my way.

(*Dennis puffs*)

It's gently dropping once more towards you.

(*It descends atop Shrew.*)

It is settling back in.

(*It rests on her face.*)

Feel it nestle into place. Feel it settle. Breathe.

(*Dennis rises, removes the filament, returns it carefully to the box, and closes it.*)

You've been able to consider yourself in the fullness of your strengths, and weaknesses, in a way that you have never before.

You feel serene. Focused. Safe. You feel *strong.*

You're *alive.* Wherever else you may be in five seconds, five minutes, five years, or five decades. Right now, *you* are most definitely here, and *you* are in charge of your life.

(*Beat.*)

Thoughts?

(*Beat*)

Mammoth   I'm not done yet.

(*Realizing that this is true.*)

I'm not done yet. I was thinking, as I was watching myself. What's my hurry? I may be finished eventually, I mean, I *will be,* eventually, we all will be. But not yet. There may be another mammoth out there, somewhere, a male, maybe another herd. It's a big world. It's possible.

Shrew   Totally possible.

Mammoth   I'll keep searching. Why not? What have I got to lose?

Is that silly?

Dennis   No.

Shrew   No. That's great.

And when you find him?

Mammoth   And when I find him?

When I find him? I'll laugh. Cry, maybe. Almost certainly cry. And then there is going to be some serious, *serious* lovemaking.

T Rex	I don't know yet what I'll do. But I'll be back next session to find out.
Glen	Same.
Dennis	What about you?
Smallpox	I need to apologize.
Dennis	To whom?
Smallpox	To all of you. I needed to believe that I would exist forever. I clung jealously to that notion and now I understand that I won't, no more than that tiny mote of suspended gossamer will. I confess, I have been tormented by the terrible, inescapable inequality of it. I can see that someday I will not exist and have been absolutely wracked that perhaps *he* will. But now I realize and accept that extinction is universal and there is a sublime, transcendent impartiality to it all. Eventually, everything, everything including *this* useless sticky strand of DNA will be expunged. We will all be annihilated and when that happens…When that happens we will all be gathered together in the glorious expansive brotherhood of obliteration.
Dennis	And that satisfies you?
Smallpox	Immensely.
Dennis	Good. Any other thoughts?
	None?
	We can take a break.
	(*The others leave the group, but Shrew remains with Dennis.*)
T Rex	That rhythmic breathing has made me so *thirsty*.

Mammoth	Me too. I'm parched.
	(*Dennis and Shrew are left alone.*)
Dennis	You're not going out to stretch your legs?
Shrew	No.
Dennis	I see.
	(*sits*)
	You didn't say much after our exercise.
Shrew	I still don't feel better.
Dennis	Well. You know, it's not really possible for me to *make you* feel better.
Shrew	Tell me what to do. Tell me how to find some kind of peace.
Dennis	If I knew how to make everyone magically feel good, I would. I can't. I don't think anyone has that power. In the end, I'm just an instrument.
	So, I can't tell you that.
Shrew	Who can?
Dennis	Only you can deal with the fundamental problem.
Shrew	But what is it?
Dennis	To live as though there will never be another moment. To live as long as you are able to live.
Shrew	And when my time comes?
Dennis	You will breathe each breath knowing that you have truly lived.
Shrew	And when I can't breathe any longer?
Dennis	You will close your eyes and rest. And it will be the sweetest most restful rest of your life.
	(*Beat.*)
Shrew	Maybe you are an instrument. Maybe I am

an instrument too, and perhaps when the deity finishes with us, when she has used us completely and we are too scarred and infirm, she licks all our bloody spots off, and when we are finally clean, she reclaims us and returns us to infinity.

(*Mammoth peeks her head in.*)

Mammoth   We're just coming back in.

Smallpox   (*From behind her*) Can you *try* not to brush against everything? The hairs cling.

Mammoth   Oh!

Smallpox   (*To Dennis*) Do you have any Scotch tape that can be used to pick up strays?

Dennis   I'm afraid not.

Shrew   (*Touching Dennis on the arm and rising*) I'm just going to grab some water. (*To Dennis, looking him in the eye.*) It's time. Goodbye.

Dennis   Goodbye.

(*Dennis observes Shrew as she exits.*)

Mammoth   You keep bothering me about shedding hairs and I will climb right up on top of you, and you will be removing hairs till this time next century.

Smallpox   If you had a vacuum positioned here by the doorway we could run it over her before she enters.

Mammoth   Can we begin?

T Rex   We better wait for Shrew.

Mammoth   She went to get water.

Dennis   She didn't get any water.

Mammoth   She didn't?

Dennis   No.

	(*Slight beat.*)
All	Ohh.
Mammoth	I'll miss her.
Dennis	Everyone.
	I'm afraid, that something has come up and we'll have to cut our time together short.
Mammoth	Aw.
T Rex	Aw.
Dennis	My apologies for the short notice. And a replacement will be taking the next session.
T Rex	How will we know when—
Dennis	You will each be contacted. I thought we had a very fruitful go round this evening. Thank you for your patience, generosity, and candor. Once again, you have been inspirational.
Mammoth	It was a great session.
T Rex	Thank you.
Dennis	Come together.
	Ready?
	(*And, once everyone is holding hands, they sing.*)
All	We are often tossed and driven on the restless sea of time; somber skies and howling tempests oft succeed a bright sunshine; in that land of perfect day, when the mists have rolled away, we will understand it better by and by.
	(*They release hands.*)
	Good evening, everybody.
	(*Everyone begins to exit.*)
Dennis	Glen, not you.

	(*Glen stops.*)
	Can you please stay behind?
Mammoth	Good night.
Dennis	Good night.
Smallpox	Good night.
	(*As he goes out the door.*)
T Rex	We're going for drinks around the corner if you want to join.
Smallpox	Yes, you must come.
Glen	All right.
Mammoth	(*Off stage, as the door opens to the elements.*) It's raining!
T Rex	(*Off stage*) I'll leave a note with the address. (*The office door closes with a click, and they're all gone with the exception of Glen and Dennis.*)
Glen	Yes?
Dennis	This will be your final session with me.
Glen	Why? Is there something I've done?
Dennis	No, it's just— (*Joan opens the door and enters.*)
Joan	Dennis? Oh, excuse me, the door was open, so I thought… (*Seeing Glen*) Wait. What's going on? (*To Dennis*) What are you doing?
Dennis	You can't just barge in—
Joan	(*To Glen*) You shouldn't be here.
Glen	Did you tell her?
Dennis	No.

Joan	Tell me what? (*To Dennis*) How dare you.
Dennis	How dare I?
Joan	Are you offering him therapy?
Dennis	Well, obviously.
Joan	Really?
Dennis	I have a responsibility—
Joan	That's a clear breach—
Dennis	Breach? *You* are one to speak of breach—
Joan	—and a conflict of interest.
Dennis	—He came to me.
Joan	—Yes, and he came to me as well.
Glen	You mentioned to me one time that your husband was a talented therapist, and I've found him—
Joan	(*To Glen*) Shut up. (*To Dennis*) So you just permitted the sessions to continue to see how far it would go?
Dennis	I continued sessions as needed and required. Of course, I didn't know the exact situation when he first requested my services.
Glen	This is awkward. (*Pause.*)
Joan	If it's helpful to know, we're finished he and I.
Glen	We are?
Joan	Yes, of course.
Glen	When did you decide we were finished?
Joan	Almost immediately. Have we seen each other in months? Or phoned? Did I return any of your calls?
Glen	No, but I didn't see that as a deal breaker.

Joan	Dennis.
Dennis	Don't.
Joan	You learned today, didn't you?
Glen	No, he learned, ah, weeks ago.
Joan	Can you *stop*? We're talking about something different.
Glen	(*confused*) Wait. What *are* we talking about?
Joan	Tell him.
Dennis	Is it necessary to bring him—
Joan	*Tell* him.
Dennis	Five years ago I had a melanoma surgically removed, but not before it had metastasized to my lungs. I discovered today that it has spread to my liver, bones and… the long and short of it is, it's inoperable. I was informed that I probably have weeks, not months.
Glen	Ohhh.

(*After performing some internal calculations, then to Joan.*)

So, when you say we're finished…?

Joan	No, Glen we're finished. I won't be seeing you again.
Glen	Okay. Well. Looks like you two have things to work out.

(*He attempts to walk away.*)

Dennis	Glen.
Glen	What?
Dennis	What I intended to say to you. This is the last opportunity we will have to speak. Don't wait. Time's running out, but change is still possible.
Glen	Right.

Dennis	At a certain point, waiting isn't an option.
Glen	(*Slight pause*) Right.
	(*Glen exits.*)
Joan	(*Looking after Glen as he exits*) It was never an important—
Dennis	Don't.
Joan	It was just a—
	It was a, surprisingly bad choice.
	And it never, ever occurred to me that he would approach you.
Dennis	I thought about dismissing him when I found out, but…
	(*Beat*)
Joan	The nurse called me. She was concerned from your reaction…
	You should have told me.
Dennis	As you know I only found out this morning.
Joan	When you first suspected.
Dennis	I *always* suspected things were getting worse.
	I always hoped I was wrong.
	I didn't want to worry you.
Joan	You didn't want me to be part of it.
Dennis	No, no, that's not it.
Joan	Yes, yes it was, that was it exactly. From the instant you were first diagnosed, you pushed me out.
Dennis	I didn't push you out -
Joan	You most certainly did, you didn't want me there—
Dennis	*Of course,* I didn't want you there—
Joan	—you wanted to hold onto it. You wanted to control it.

Dennis	*Of course,* I wanted to control it—who doesn't want to control their illness?
Joan	You should have made space for me.
Dennis	I didn't know how. I didn't know how to make space for *me*—
Joan	You share things in a relationship.
Dennis	Not that.
Joan	*Everything.*
Dennis	No.
Joan	*Everything.* You share everything in a relationship, you share your successes, your disappointments, you share your sickness.
Dennis	Ohmygod, who wants to share that? Appointments, ointments, x-rays, clammy waiting rooms, endless inspections, injections, unsightly rashes, tubes and pills and all those terrible, awful, peppy ads, people with gleaming smiles promoting their plucky fight against cancer, what incredible bone-headed bullshit! I don't feel *plucky.*
	I feel like the world is an enormous sheet of sandpaper that is every day wearing me down a little bit more. I'm raw. I'm this thin. Paper thin. I few more rubs, I'd be gone. I was scared. And wrong. Wrong to exclude you. Come back.
Joan	I can help care for you.
Dennis	I don't want you to care for me. I don't want you to turn my sheets and cook my meals, I can hire someone to do that.
Joan	What do you want?
Dennis	Move in.
Joan	And do what?

Dennis	Live with me.
Joan	When?
Dennis	Now. Come live with me now.
Joan	You said you wanted to—
Dennis	—handle things.
Joan	You said you needed—
Dennis	—space.
	Yes. I thought I would have time to fix things. I thought I could do things one after another—resolve my health issues first, then repair our relationship.
	I couldn't figure out how to do both at the same time.
	(*They hold hands.*)
	I was frightened. But I always loved you.
Joan	What was our problem?
Dennis	It was the sickness, and the medication, and the same old problem as always. Me.
	(*Beat.*)
Joan	If I come back, we'll run into the same difficulties.
Dennis	No, we won't. I can change.
Joan	There's no time anymore.
Dennis	Well, exactly. I know I can change because I won't have to do it for long.
	(*She thumps him on the chest.*)
Joan	Why couldn't we get along?
Dennis	Well. We did, for a long time, then we didn't, and none of that matters anymore. Here we are.
Joan	If you want me to come back, you have to come back too.

Dennis	What does that mean?
Joan	I can't return just to wait for you to die. You understand that? You'll have to meet me halfway.
Dennis	I'm just telling you what the doctors have told—
Joan	Screw that—stop saying weeks this and weeks that.
	(*Beat*)
Dennis	At some point, I'll die.
Joan	At *some point*, you don't know when.
Dennis	The doctors—
Joan	—Don't know either, nobody knows. It's a mystery. And you have to promise me that while I live with you, you are *living* with me. Not waiting.
	Promise me.
	(*Slight beat*)
Dennis	And if it's only a month?
Joan	Then we will have lived a month, but it could be five, or ten, and we will make every minute count, so it'll feel longer. It'll be like dog years.
Dennis	Okay.
Joan	Promise.
Dennis	I can pinky swear, if you'd like.
Joan	And screw that too.
	(*She kisses him. They continue kissing until they collapse on the floor in front of the desk. They recover, and sit with their backs against the desk.*)
	I'll move in tonight. Let me get my things.
Dennis	Make it for six, we can have a dinner function.

Joan	How will you know? Where's your precious clock?
Dennis	I chucked it. You were right about that too, I was never any good at fixing machines.

I dreamt that your precious Jesus arrived at our house, dressed in workmen's overalls. I asked him, why are you here? Have you come to heal me?

He said, no, I have come to fix your clock.

I hang my head. I have been working on it for many, many weeks, I tell him it is unfixable.

He reaches down and I see that he is wearing an enormous toolbelt, and on it are an infinity of the tiniest of instruments. And I just know, that there is one in there that could fix my broken heart if I let it, one that could heal all the hurts of any soul.

And he selects a truly, truly minute instrument, only as big as a grass blade, and he bends over the clock, and it snaps together and is repaired and right away the hands on the face of the clock begin rotating backwards, and I look up at the sky, and the stars are moving backwards as well. And he turns to me.

Now, he says. You have only this time.

(*Lights dim to black.*)

The End

THE EXTINCTION THERAPIST

An Optional Epilogue

Acts One and Two are intended to stand alone, but this epilogue may be offered as a value-added adjunct, at a later time in the run of the production at the discretion of the theatre.)

Cast

A female Woolly Mammoth—warm and expansive. A lover, not a fighter.

The Smallpox Virus—male, pale faced, arms wrapped in a strait jacket, cold and imposing. Sees himself as an Alpha.

Tyrannosaurus Rex—male, possessing an immense head and tiny forearms. Experiences anxiety issues.

An Anglerfish—both male and female of the species, the male aspect mild and unassuming, his female aspect, larger, more vibrant, dynamic, intimidating. (Should be double-cast with either Shrew or Dennis).

Glen Merrick—The charming-despite-himself Minister for the Environment, male, should perhaps remind one of a young John F. Kennedy. Early forties.

Settings

The action of the epilogue occurs in the Last Stop Bar and Grill, a shady, suspect, out-of-the-way tavern catering solely to clients approaching extinction.

	A neon sign sizzles, crackles to life and lights up, reading **The Last Stop Bar & Grill**. *Glen opens a door and steps into the bar. He closes the door, brushes the rain from his clothes, and looks about.*
T Rex	(*turning*) You found it.
Glen	(*Seeing T Rex)* Oh hi.
	It's packed.
T Rex	There's a table saved for us.
	(*Lights rise on a table.)*
	Mammoth is fetching drinks.
Smallpox	Hang your coat up, you're dripping everywhere.
Mammoth	Drinks! (*Surprised to see Glen)* Oh, you came.
Glen	I've never seen a place like this before.
T Rex	And never will again. The Last Stop Bar and Grill; a drinking establishment devoted exclusively to those on the edge of extinction. Their motto: (*Lifting a coaster from a table and reading.)* when you're dying for a drink, stop in.
Glen	You know all the, ah, regulars?
Mammoth	Pretty well.
T Rex	The usual suspects.
	(*Scans the room.*)
Mammoth	White Rumped Vulture, there.
	Darwin's fox. Glyptodon at the far table.
	Southern Cassowary, Saiga Antelope, Gharial Crocodile, Pygmy Hippo.
T Rex	Is that who I think it is beside them?
Mammoth	Eastern Black Rhino.
Mammoth &	
T Rex	Ohhh
Glen	What?

Mammoth	A shell of her former self.
T Rex	Ever since her cousin the Western Black Rhino passed, she's been fading.
	(*Anglerfish appears with more drinks.*)
Angler	But—no room for regrets or apologies.
	(*Fills the table with drinks. T Rex grabs a mug and a spoon, taps the mug.*)
T Rex	Everyone. Everyone!
	A novice has entered and wishes to pledge.
Mammoth	(*whispering to Glen*) You're a first timer here.
T Rex	Call to order.
All	Order.
Mammoth	(*whispering to Glen*) It's what they do with all the newbies.
T Rex	Sound the clarion.
All	Sounding the clarion.
	(*Mammoth employs her trunk to sound a trumpeting call.*)
T Rex	Master At No Arms—present the novice.
	(*Smallpox nudges Glen ahead.*)
	Behold the novice.
All	Beholding the novice.
T Rex	Approach the alter.
	Are you pure of heart?
Glen	Ah, no.
T Rex	Excellent, you are in good company.
	Ring the Radiant Bell.
All	Ringing the Radiant Bell.
	(*Holding a spoon in her trunk, Mammoth strikes a glass that T Rex is holding, producing a bell like peal.*)
T Rex	Has the novice been blessed?

	(*Mammoth dips her trunk into the drink and sprinkles Glen.*)
All	He has.
T Rex	Has he been baptized?
	(*Mammoth tosses the rest of the drink in his face.*)
All	He has.
Angler	Libations to the eastern horizon.
	(*A drink is passed to the individual on the right. They sip.*)
Mammoth	Libations to the western horizon.
	(*A drink is passed the individual on the left. They sip.*)
T Rex	Novice! Do you honour the setting sun, the dying candle, the retreating tide, the final quadrant of the failing moon?
	(*Mammoth nudges him.*)
Glen	I do.
Mammoth	Do you vow to respect fellow members, to stiffen your spine and swear to never, ever betray the pain, sacrifice and sacred ideals of this most Benevolent Order of the Last Stop Bar and Grill?
Glen	I do.
All	Aroo Aroo Aroo
	(*Mammoth trumpets once again*)
T Rex	Kneel.
	Present the chalice.
	(*Mammoth fills an immense tumbler with whiskey. Glen drinks from it.*)
T Rex	Stand.
	(*Glen stands*)

The Order welcomes all travellers who find
themselves standing upon a platform, having
been presented their one way no-return
ticket. The Order embraces you in the spirit of
fellowship of our universal mortality.

Prepare the novice.

(*He is presented a butter knife.*)

The saber.

All	To sever all connections with the past.
T Rex	The princely crown.

(*A basket that had previously held the salt and
pepper shaker on the table, is deployed as a
crown and placed on Glen's head.*)

All	To acknowledge the regal and sacred mystery of evanescence.
T Rex	Novice
All	Live with integrity.
T Rex	Die
All	Die
T Rex	—with dignity, knowing that
All	all things are ephemeral.
T Rex	Seek
All	Stillness.
T Rex	Embrace
All	Infinity
T Rex	And always
All	Always
T Rex	Always
	Pay your tab.
	Do you so pledge?
Glen	I do.

T Rex	I do induct you into the most Righteous, Benevolent Order, with all its attending powers, privileges, and daunting responsibilities.
	(*Mammoth trumpets. All those participating in the ritual raise a glass.*)
T Rex	Bottoms up!
All	Bottoms up!
	(*All drink and slam the emptied glasses down on the tabletop.*)
T-Rex	God that's good! Why didn't we ever invent fifteen-year-old scotch?
Mammoth	No opposable thumbs.
	(*Smallpox nods at the drinks on the table indicating he wants one. Angler holds a glass to Smallpox's mouth.*)
Smallpox	We should change the initiation.
	(*Drinks*)
	Some of the best of us don't have a backbone.
	(*Drinks*)
	Backbones are *so* overrated.
T Rex	(*To Mammoth*) What are you looking for?
Angler	(*To Glen*) Go ahead, help yourself to another.
Glen	(*Taking a glass*) Thanks.
Mammoth	I heard Pacific Mastodon stopped by not long ago.
	Not really my type.
	(*To Glen*) They're a bit short.
	But.
	(*Drinks*)
Glen	I don't see anyone like me—
Smallpox	'Like me.' Like *me*. Will you stop?? Shouldn't it be abundantly apparent at this point that

it's not all about you and those that *look like* you? Isn't it bad enough that I have had to sit through therapy tolerating your endless, tiresome, whining, mendacity, and transparent narcissism, that I have to put up with your unrelenting consummate *bullshit* here as well?

Mammoth	Be civil!
T Rex	Stay calm or they'll cut us off and throw us out.
Mammoth	Again. (*to Glen*) Last time he went on a rant, the owners refused to serve us.
Smallpox	Sorry.
All	Oooh!

No apologies!

(*They begin to chant.*)

Shooter, shooter, shooter, shooter.

Angler	Here.

(*He places a straw in the glass.*)

Smallpox	Please.

(*He bends over and plucks up the straw with his teeth and spits it out.*)

Straws are for amateurs.

Angler	Suit yourself.

(*Smallpox swiftly dips his head to table level, grasps the glass between his teeth, straightens up, downs the shot, and then tosses the empty glass to the table.*)

Smallpox	Ahh!

(*Spectators applaud.*)

Angler	You're not bothered by him, I hope.
Glen	No, no.

Angler	It's actually insecurity that prompts his prickly attitude.
Glen	I'm used to it. As a politician you develop a thick skin.
Smallpox	Oh yes, in therapy he has been the very model of charity and tolerance and turning the other cheek.
	(*Mammoth brings over a tray of shooters.*)
Mammoth	I'll fetch us pretzels.
T Rex	And jerky. Get jerky.
	(*Not receiving a response, he stands*)
	Jerky!
	Always gotta get it myself. You want jerky?
Angler	Sure.
T Rex	Never send a vegetarian for snacks.
Angler	Cheers.
Glen	Cheers.
	(*They drink.*)
	Um, who are you?
Angler	Anglerfish.
Glen	Really?
Angler	Really.
	You sound surprised.
Glen	I always envisioned you as being…bigger. More teeth.
Mammoth	(*Rejoining the group*) You're—
	Pretzel?
	(*Glen takes some.*)
	—thinking of the female of the species.
	(*Places snacks on the table.*)
	Everyone makes that mistake.

Angler	Sexual dimorphism. Makes quite a difference in presentation.
Glen	Ah. So, you're (*he gestures to the Tavern's sign*) in trouble too.
Angler	I prefer not to call it trouble.
Glen	Oh. What do you call it?
Angler	Destiny. And everyone has one.
Glen	Oh. I'm surprised to learn you're experiencing, this particular destiny.
Angler	Why?
Glen	From my sketchy recollection—
	(*T Rex returns with a platter of jerky.*)
T Rex	Some? Lovely smoky flavor.
Glen	—derived from a single old national geographic article I browsed in a dentist's washroom, you're kind of off the beaten path. Live off on your own, a long way down.
Angler	A long way down?
Glen	In the ocean. Deep.
Angler	(*Plucks an ice cube from his water glass and flicks it into Glen's drink*)
	Is that chilling just the top section or the entire drink?
	Thanks to humans, the oceans are warming, my friend, and they warm all the way down.
Smallpox	*Humans!*
	(*He grabs another shooter between his teeth, drinks it and tosses the glass aside.*)
Mammoth	(*More to herself than anyone else.*) Oh no.
T Rex	Now really, there's no point in raising a fuss, calm yourself—
Smallpox	Humans hunger to control me—

T Rex	(*To himself*) Here we go.
Smallpox	—but their appetites are too great, they hang on, vainly hoping that the moment will emerge when they may employ me safely. But there is no safety.
	(*He grasps another drink in his teeth, gulps it down, tosses it aside.*)
	There *is no safety!* I cannot be quelled, cannot be tamed, cannot be vanquished! I will rise again. Rise again! And this time nothing will quench my thirst, no drink that will temper the terrible, terrible *heat!*
	(*And then, abruptly, he passes out, crashing to the table, face first. Mammoth pulls the snacks out of the way just in time, but Smallpox has upended some drinks.*)
T Rex	(*Brushing himself off*) Man, he *sucks* as a drinking partner!
Mammoth	(*Brushing herself off*) *Every* time he comes here it's the same.
Angler	(*Rising to get a cloth*) Can you lift him?
T Rex	It's always the biggest who has to lift the big, drunken, dead weight.
	(*He raises Smallpox. Angler returns with a cloth and mops up the spill.*)
Mammoth	Why can't he demonstrate a smidgen of self-restraint?
T Rex	I suppose that's the thing about a successful plague—
	(*He lowers Smallpox*)
	—they never understand moderation.
Angler	"I cannot be prevented from knocking over

the drinks and making a total mess" is more like it. Lift your glass.

(*Glen lifts his drink, and Angler cleans there as well.*)

Mammoth	I'm going to fetch paper towels.
	(*She exits.*)
T Rex	Oooh—he spilled Scotch in the snacks.
	(*He lifts the two plates and exits. Beat. They both consider Smallpox a moment.*)
Glen	Have you ever attended therapy?
Angler	No. (*absently*)
Glen	Why not?
Angler	The only place you are ever going to learn the truth is in a bar. There, you are going to get the final truth—and the final judgment. Here, in the Benevolent Order, we strive to speak truth to power.
Glen	What power?
Angler	What power? There's only ever one power. The power of life and death. Everything that attempts to erase you is just another manifestation of that power.
	Fight the power.
Glen	Fight the power.
	(*They clink glasses and drink.*)
Glen	One thing about therapy, though—it's made me think.
Angler	Really?
Glen	Yea.
Angler	About what?
Glen	My life. My life and…
	(*He drinks.*)

	…how stuck I am.
Angler	And did you come away from your session unstuck?
Glen	Not yet.
Angler	So, you're going to do something about it today?
Glen	Well. Not this instant. Rome wasn't built in a day.
Angler	Of course not. It'd be ridiculous to try to do everything in one day.
Glen	Unrealistic.
Angler	Why not a week, when you've had a chance to think things through?
Glen	Exactly. You don't want to rush things.
T Rex	(*off stage*) Pickled eggs?
Glen	What?
T Rex	(*off stage*) You want pickled eggs? Scotch eggs?
Glen	Sure. Pickled.
	(*An amazing transformation takes place. Angler stands, unzips—*
T Rex	(*off stage*) How many?
Glen	Maybe two.
	…and from the fresh unzipped opening emerges the fins and teeth and girth and dangling signature rod of the much larger, much more dynamic, much more dangerous, wider-mouthed, sharper-toothed, curiously beguiling, Female Anglerfish.
Angler	Even a week is hurried. (*As she continues to unfurl*) Why not a month?
Glen	Sure, that might be more reasonable—

(*Mammoth returns with paper towels.*)

Angler	Why not a year? Five years? Ten? What does it matter?

(*T Rex returns with a dry plate of snacks. Glen turns and for the first time sees who is seated beside him.*)

Why change at all?

Glen	(*startled*) Sorry?
All	Shot!

(*T Rex hands a drink to Glen, who downs it.*)

Glen	Who are you? Who is she?
T Rex	The Female Angler Fish.
Mammoth	Surprises everyone. Same species, different appearance.
T Rex	We never know which one will come calling.
Angler	Which one? But of course, we are both the same.
Glen	I don't understand. Where did—
Angler	What's to understand? I am just another aspect of the individual you were addressing earlier.
Glen	Quite different looking.
Angler	We are two sides of the same metaphorical coin.
	Tiny, thin, and frail, the male sweeps the cold waters of deep oceans, sifting darkness, casting for signs and traces of pheromones indicating a female presence.
	If the male overcomes the odds, detects traces of a female's hormone, and successfully locates a partner, he quickly opens his mouth wide and latches on.
	But.

(*She drinks.*)

Everything in life comes at a cost. The very instant the male makes contact with the female is also the last truly free moment of his life. The enzymes generated on contact disintegrate the connecting tissue, of his mouth and lips. His teeth dissolve, his muscles shrivel, and skin from the female host grows over top of the parasitic male as he finally fulfills his ardent reproductive urges. Sated, at the end of his courtship, he becomes blissfully, perpetually connected as a dangling, inert, minor appendage of the more active agent.

Glen	Quite a, courtship.
Angler	You…

(*She touches Glen on his nose.*)

…remind me a little of my other half.

Glen	Well, thank you. I guess.
Angler	I imagine your life is in considerable disarray.
Glen	Well—
Angler	Don't take it as a criticism. Everyone's life at this bar is in a little disarray.

You're searching as well, aren't you?

Glen	After a fashion.
Angler	Laden with regrets.
Glen	Everyone has regrets.
Angler	You feel disappointment.
Glen	Sure.
Angler	You're anxious.
Glen	Certainly anxious.
Angler	You feel lost.

	Inadequate.
	Disposable.
	(*Suddenly intense*) And yet, you desire!
	You desire so many things!
	You know what you must do? Do you?
	Do you?
Glen	(*slightly frightened*) No, what?
Angler	Karaoke!
All	Karaoke! Whoooo! (*Celebration*)
Angler	(*To the others*) What shall it be?
T Rex	Every Rose Has Its Thorn?
Mammoth	We did that last time!
T Rex	What do you want?
Mammoth	Sultans of Swing!
Angler	No! How about Foo Fighters' Everlong?
T Rex	Nooo! Everlong is too f-ing ever long!
Mammoth	Let's go with the classics, then.
T Rex	Dust in the Wind?
Angler	Sympathy for the Devil?
Mammoth, Angler, T Rex	*Hotel California!*
	(*They all immediately commence wordlessly 'singing' along with the final guitar solo of Hotel California, and somehow produce a strange, but curiously—eerily—satisfying, harmony. They finish. Beat.*)
Glen	What kind of karaoke is that?
T Rex	In The Last Stop Bar and Grill, only the final wordless, musical refrain of a song is honoured.
Mammoth	There are a number that are very popular.

Angler	Based on length.
T Rex	Complexity.
Mammoth	And passion.
T Rex	The dying final notes of the Stone's "Miss You" receives a lot of requests.
All	(*Demonstrating*) Ooh ooh ooh ooh ooha ooh
T Rex	Try it.
Angler	Join in!
	(*Glen joins in with the closing instrumental of Miss You, tentatively at first, but with growing confidence.*)
All	Ooah oooah ooowa oooa ooo!
	Ooa oo, oo.
	(*They groove, and finish, gloriously, spookily.*)
Angler	A drinking game!
Glen	Okay!
Mammoth	Great!
T Rex	All right!
	(*Angler grabs pencils from the basket on the table* and *distributes them.*)
Angler	Write the answer on the bottom of your coaster, and place it face down.
	(*They all await the question, pencil in hand.*)
	Ways that you most often envision your final demise.
Glen	How is that a drinking game?
Angler	If we correctly guess your answer prior to turning over your coaster, you drink.
	(*Angler sets glasses in front of everyone, fills them.*)
	If we fail to guess it, *we* drink.
Angler	Who goes first?

T Rex	I'll go.
Angler	(*guessing*) Consumed in the white-hot flames following the explosion of a giant earth-bound asteroid.
	(*T Rex turns his coaster over. Angler's guess was correct.*)
T Rex	Right. (*He drinks.*)
Mammoth	Me next.
Angler	Alone and frozen on a barren glacier.
Mammoth	Nope.
	(*Angler drinks.*)
T Rex	A broken heart.
Mammoth	Nope.
T Rex	I thought for certain that would be it. You're sure it's not of a broken heart?
Mammoth	Nope.
	(*T Rex drinks.*)
Glen	Devoured by saber tooth tigers or, what were they called, dire wolves?
Mammoth	That's two answers, but nope and nope.
	(*Glen drinks. Mammoth turns her coaster over.*)
	Long, lingering slow starvation.
Angler	That would have been my second guess.
Glen	My turn.
Mammoth	(*guessing*) Fatality while under the influence.
Angler	Me too.
T Rex	Me too.
Glen	(*Flipping his coaster over. They are correct.*) Unfortunate drunken happenstance.
	(*He drinks*)

	Where are washrooms located?
Mammoth	That way. (*Gesturing with her trunk*)
	(*He exits.*)
	Should he be here?
T Rex	No one forced him to come.
Angler	Or to stay.
	And he certainly possesses an extraordinary capacity to drink.
Mammoth	Yes. But maybe we should just cut the evening short.
Angler	I don't think so.
T Rex	The evening will go as long as the evening needs to go.
Mammoth	I only came because I was hoping that Mastadon would show up.
	(*She nods at Smallpox*) And he's passed out—
T Rex	He'll revive.
Mammoth	Why don't we just call it a night?
Angler	Calm yourself. Life is not a catch and release affair.
	(*As Glen returns.*)
Glen	What were you talking about?
T Rex	Nothing.
Angler	Another drinking game!
	What is your most hidden secret?
Mammoth	What do you mean?
Angler	Reveal a hidden secret or take a drink.
	(*Each strives to recollect a secret.*)
T Rex	I have one.
	A secret skill. Although it's commonly assumed that because we are the largest

carnivorous reptile, our senses don't have to be very acute. We pride ourselves on excellent binocular vision.

Hold that menu open.

(*Glen holds the menu open.*)

Take a step back.

(*He steps back.*)

Farther.

(*He steps back farther. T Rex reads the bottom line.*)

Bottom line. "Chicken wings, barbecued, honey mustard, sweet and sour."

Ay?

All	Amazing.

(*They drink.*)

Smallpox	Ohhhh. My. God.

(*All turn to look at Smallpox, who slowly raises his head from the table top.*)

That is *pathetic*.

I will share a *genuine* secret with you, since you seem not to fathom what the word actually means. As you know, I presently exist, confined and isolated in two locations in all the world.

Officially.

Glen	Officially?
Smallpox	But I also exist, unofficially, and unacknowledged, elsewhere.

I survive, dormant, in the stiff, frozen corpses of the thousands who perished in the last round of plague in the nineteen hundreds and whose bodies lie buried beneath the permafrost in the far north, waiting, *waiting* for the temperature to rise. And isn't it delicious that climate change, the unintended genie conjured by humans will be the spectre that summons me back to the surface?

(Laughs, a low throaty laugh.)

That, my friends, *that* constitutes the very definition of a slow reveal. Just imagine what splendid retribution I will be able to accomplish as the world gradually warms and all those thousands of gloriously infected, frozen bodies thaw. The dead shall truly rise!

(He laughs heartily and suddenly collapses once again. His companions consider his recumbent body. Glen turns to Angler.)

Glen	You?
Angler	I am able to unhinge my jaw and devour prey twice my size.

(She unhinges it and lowers it part way, then retracts it.)

Glen	Wow.

(Beat. They drink.)

Angler	And you?
Glen	I've got nothing.
All	Oh, come on!
Glen	No, I am Secretless Joe.

(He drinks instead of offering secret.)

Tried to think of something. Came up blank.

(He pours another drink, his hand is unsteady, and he pours on the table. Angler shifts his hand so that he is once again pouring into his glass.)

Whoops.

> Anything approaching a dark secret I already shared in group. I'm purged, cleansed, expunged of my x-rated material.

(*He consumes the entire glass, and makes to pour another. Mammoth takes the bottle from him.*)

Mammoth   Maybe you should go home, get a—

T Rex   (*interrupting*) You want to play Eight Ball?

Mammoth   Is a table free?

T Rex   The Bornean Orangutan and Giant Otter just left.

(Angler *nudges her in the direction of the table.*)

Angler   You two go.

(*They exit, leaving Angler and Glen alone with the recumbent, passed out Smallpox. Angler gestures to Mammoth and T Rex as they go.*)

They won't be gone long. In the Last Stop Bar and Grill, Eight Ball is played only with the final eponymous ball of the Game, the Eight Ball.

Still, T Rex having those tiny forearms presents a bit of a handicap.

Glen   I can only imagine.

(*Beat. Smallpox snores. Angler fills Glen's glass to the brim.*)

Angler   No point in moderation now. Cheers.

Glen   Cheers.

(*They drink. At this juncture it's clear that Glen is quite drunk. Angler leans in.*)

Angler   So, what is it?

Glen   What is what?

Angler   Your secret.

Glen	Oh. Nothing.
Angler	*Everyone* has a secret.
Glen	I've got zip.
Angler	Come on.
	(*She pours him another drink.*)
	You can do it.
	(*Beat*)
Glen	All right.
Angler	I knew it!
Glen	But it's boring.
Angler	I'm all ears.
Glen	In group, we talked about, my challenge. The therapist told me I had painted myself into a corner.
Angler	And?
Glen	Advised me not to hesitate. Told me to use my time to 'get out'.
	(*He drinks.*)
Angler	But?
Glen	But, there is no way out. I've tried. It was the only reason I attended the group in the first place, but at a certain point you discover life is nothing but corners.
Angler	It is written in the Book of Fate, that there is always a way out.
Glen	The Book of Fate.
	(*Takes a drink.*)
	Never read that book, myself. And wouldn't have thought you had an opportunity to read much down there in the deep, dark, depths.
Angler	But you forget, I have my own nightlight.

(Click, the light dangling from her head winks on.)

Glen (*Momentarily arrested by it.*) That's interesting.

Angler (*The light sways and bobs*) My signature element, a beacon used to draw creatures to their final exit.

It's beautiful, isn't it?

Glen Curiously compelling.

(All other lights of the bar slowly begin dimming. T Rex returns.)

Glen Oh, you're back.

Angler Where's Mammoth?

T Rex I helped her find Mastodon.

Angler And now novice, time for judgment.

Glen Judgment?

Angler You pledged not to betray your fellows.

T Rex But you already have.

Glen What are you talking about, who have I betrayed?

Angler Who have you not betrayed?

T Rex An entire world of betrayal, right there.

(Glen turns and views the bar and all the clients.)

Look at them all attending their extinction.

Glen Wait, wait.

(He turns and considers T Rex who is clearly blocking Glen's exit.)

Wait.

(He turns to face Angler once again.)

I thought I was joining a benevolent order.

T Rex	It *is* a benevolent order.
Angler	The most benevolent order. What could be more benevolent than to be corrected for error?
T Rex	And you are called to account.
Angler	Do you have anything to say in your defense?
Glen	I—
T Rex	—Although there is scarcely anything you can say.
Glen	I don't know…I don't even know what I'm charged with.
Angler	That's all right. Your confession already condemns you.
Glen	What confession? I thought I was a member. You made me a member.
Angler	It is your membership that condemns you. Don't you understand? No one who is a member is fated to live.
Glen	I resign my membership then.
Angler	Membership is irrevocable.
Glen	I've offended you. I see that now and apologize.
T Rex	Your apology is irredeemable.
Angler	And your hesitation condemns you.
T Rex	No one who actually wished to save others would delay taking action.
Glen	I don't know what to say.
T Rex	You have said everything that needed saying. Here and elsewhere.
Glen	You mean about my job? I was ineffective in my job, yes, maybe I took a few liberties. Should have tried to—

Angler	How say you?
T Rex	Guilty as charged.
Glen	That's hardly fair.
Angler	Wake up the Master Of No Arms.
T Rex	Wake up!
	(*He jostles the dozing Smallpox. Glen turns to depart, but T Rex steps in front of him. Glen turns in the other direction. Smallpox rises and impedes Glen's exit.*)
Smallpox	What?
Angler	Was there ever anyone you extinguished who desired to perish?
Smallpox	Never.
Angler	And yet, was there ever anyone who didn't deserve their fate?
Smallpox	Never.
Glen	*He's* hardly objective.
Angler	Having viewed a representative sample of millions, he surely holds an educated opinion, wouldn't you say?
	(*T Rex and Smallpox move closer to Glen.*)
Glen	I wouldn't have come here.
	(*He tries to leave but is pushed back toward Angler.*)
	I wouldn't have come here if I'd known that I would be questioned like this.
Angler	You would not be here if you could be anywhere else.
Smallpox	You made your decision.
T Rex	Just as you made your decisions that condemned others.
Glen	What decisions? I didn't make decisions.

Smallpox	And *that* is what condemns you.
T Rex	Not making a decision, is in itself a decision.
Smallpox	All your thousands of indecisions constituting a single stinging condemnation.
Angler	All your thousands of indecisions manifestly condemning others.
Glen	I might have been wrong from time to time, but who isn't?
Angler	Relativism is the excuse of the weak.
Smallpox	Either you were wrong, or you weren't.
T Rex	Were you?
	(*Steps closer.*)
Smallpox	Or weren't you?
	(*Steps closer.*)
Angler	Were you?
	(*T Rex pushes Glen toward Angler.*)
Smallpox	Or weren't you?
	(*Smallpox pushes Glen toward Angler.*)
Glen	*Some of the time!*
	(*Fighting free for a moment.*)
	Surely, some of the time is forgivable.
Angler	There is no forgiveness in obliteration. Forgiveness is what the living give the living. Those who can expect nothing but death have no capacity to forgive the living, and those that are no longer living can no longer accept that gift.
	(*T Rex pushes Glen closer to Angler.*)
Glen	But there were reasons.
	(*Smallpox shoves Glen closer to Angler*)
Smallpox	We have no interest in reasons.

Angler	What are reasons? Words received in lieu of actions. Words provided where actions have failed. Reasons are copper payment for an invoice that insists upon the gold currency of deeds. And your tab is due.

(The light that dangles from her head brightens at the same time that the rest of the lights on stage continue to dim.)

Glen   I'm sorry!

T Rex   Take a shot.

(He snatches a drink from the table and thrusts it in Glen's mouth.

The only light illuminating the bar now is the one dangling from Angler's head. The only images remaining are of Angler's dreadful gaping mouth, her dangling light and the face of the hapless Glen. Moment of silence.)

Angler   Come a little closer.

(Her jaws slowly unhinge and open to their terrifying fullest capacity—Lights out. The startling sound of the jaws snapping shut is heard, and a scream. Then in the dark, T Rex and Smallpox join Angler for the dying final refrain of Miss You.)

All Three   Ooooh ooooh oooh

Ooooh ooooh oooh

Ooooh

(The Stone's version rises behind them, louder, and...

(The End.)

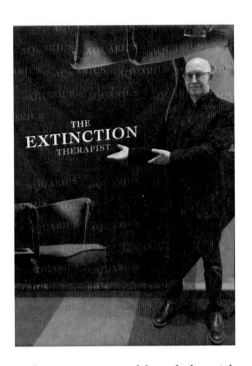

Professor Clem Martini is a celebrated playwright, novelist, and screenwriter with over thirty plays and thirteen books of fiction and non-fiction to his credit. His text on playwriting, *The Blunt Playwright* is employed by colleges and universities across the country. His books include *Upside Down: A Family's Journey Through Mental Illness*, the W.O. Mitchell Award-winning *Bitter Medicine: A Graphic Memoir of Mental Illness* and the Alberta Trade Non-Fiction Book of the Year Award-winning, *The Unravelling*. A passionate advocate on behalf of issues associated with suicide, mental-illness-related-stigma, and family care giving, Clem was a member of the Canadian Mental Health Commission, and has been an invited speaker at a number of conferences, symposia and health related gatherings. He is a Fellow of The Royal Society of Canada, a recipient of the ATB Financial Healing through the Arts Award, and a Professor of Drama in the School of Creative and Performing Arts at the University of Calgary.